EASY DIABETIC RECIPES

Publications International, Ltd.

Pictured on the front cover *(clockwise from top right):* Frozen Berry Pops *(page 173),* Buffalo Cauliflower Bites *(page 14)* and Chopped Roasted Chicken Salad *(page 156).*

Pictured on the back cover *(clockwise from top left):* Mini Meatloaves *(page 86),* Butternut Squash Oven Fries *(page 112),* and Peach-Melba Shortcakes *(page 176).*

Photographs on front cover *(top right and bottom left)*, and pages 157 and 172 © Shutterstock.com.

ISBN: 978-1-64558-603-6

Manufactured in China.

8 7 6 5 4 3 2 1

Microwave Cooking: Microwave ovens vary in wattage. Use the cooking times as guidelines and check for doneness before adding more time. ̄

Nutritional Analysis: Every effort has been made to check the accuracy of the nutritional information that appears with each recipe. However, because numerous variables account for a wide range of values for certain foods, nutritive analyses in this book should be considered approximate.

WARNING: Food preparation, baking and cooking involve inherent dangers: misuse of electric products, sharp electric tools, boiling water, hot stoves, allergic reactions, foodborne illnesses and the like, pose numerous potential risks. Publications International, Ltd. (PIL) assumes no responsibility or liability for any damages you may experience as a result of following recipes, instructions, tips or advice in this publication.

While we hope this publication helps you find new ways to eat delicious foods, you may not always achieve the results desired due to variations in ingredients, cooking temperatures, typos, errors, omissions or individual cooking abilities.

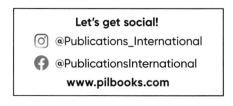

Let's get social!

@Publications_International

@PublicationsInternational

www.pilbooks.com

CONTENTS

INTRODUCTION

WHAT IS DIABETES?

Millions of people today either may have diabetes or are at risk for the getting diabetes. Although there is currently no cure for the disease, it is very treatable. You can easily live a long and healthy life by understanding diabetes and taking care of yourself.

To get the most from the latest advances in diabetes care, you need to understand just what it means to have diabetes. A good place to start is learning how the body uses fuel and how that process goes awry in diabetes.

EDUCATING YOURSELF

You've probably already heard the word glucose. It is an important player in the body and in diabetes. In your bloodstream, circulating to all your body parts, is sugar. Most of the sugar in your bloodstream is the kind called glucose. Glucose's main job is to supply the body's cells with energy. Glucose is a quickly available fuel used by nearly all tissues in the body, and it's the only fuel your brain and nerves can use. The brain can survive without glucose for only a short time. Therefore, your brain directs your body to protect your glucose level, making sure it does not fall too low. It does this by increasing the production of certain hormones. These hormones cause the liver to release its stored-up sugar into the bloodstream. So, when people talk about blood sugar, they are really talking about glucose.

The glucose in your body comes from three major nutrients: fat, protein, and carbohydrate. About 10 percent of the fat and 50 percent of the protein you eat is eventually converted into glucose (the rest is used for other purposes or stored in the body's fat cells), but nearly 100 percent of the carbohydrate you eat is broken down into glucose. Chewing and swallowing begin the digestive process of breaking down starches and larger sugar molecules into glucose. The enzymes in your mouth and your intestines complete the breakdown. The glucose is then absorbed into the bloodstream and travels throughout the body. That's when the pancreas plays a vital role.

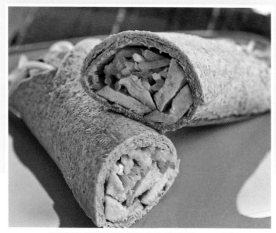

GRILLED BUFFALO CHICKEN WRAPS, page 37

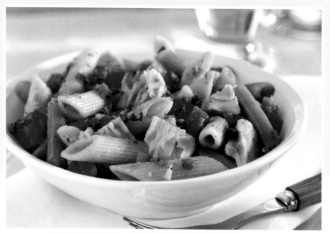

PASTA WITH TUNA, GREEN BEANS & TOMATOES, page 64

The pancreas is a fist-size organ just behind your stomach. One of its jobs is to make enzymes for food digestion. But the pancreas also plays another important role. It contains small groups of cells, the islets of Langerhans, that make hormones, which are released into your bloodstream. Some 80 percent of these islet cells are called "beta" cells that make two hormones: amylin and insulin. Amylin plays a secondary role in regulating appetite and the rate of digestion. Insulin plays a major role in allowing the body's cells to take in proteins, fatty acids, and glucose. Insulin is like a key that opens a door to the body's cells, so the nutrients needed by the cells can get inside. When a person who does not have diabetes eats any food, their blood glucose levels rises. The beta cells detect this rise and release more insulin. The insulin goes to the liver, telling the liver to make less glucose. It also helps the liver, muscle, and fat cells to take up more glucose. This allows nutrients from the recently eaten food to enter and "feed" the body's cells, it keeps blood glucose from rising too high even after eating, and it allows the glucose level to return to a normal, healthy range quickly. When we go many hours without eating, such as between meals or during sleep, the insulin levels fall, causing the liver to make more glucose to provide energy for the brain, heart, lungs, etc, until the next meal.

In a person with diabetes, this process doesn't work properly. Either the beta cells have lost the ability to produce insulin or the insulin does not do its job as well as it should. As a result, the amount of glucose in the blood rises and the body's cells become deprived of the fuel they need.

DIFFERENT TYPES OF DIABETES

There are three major types of diabetes: type 1 diabetes, type 2 diabetes, and gestational diabetes. Each type requires a different type of treatment.

TYPE 1 DIABETES

This type affects about 5 percent of all people with diabetes. It is sometimes referred to as juvenile diabetes, because there is a higher rate of diagnosis in children, but people of any age can develop type 1 diabetes. It may also be called insulin-dependent diabetes, because those with type 1 diabetes require insulin (via injections or an insulin pump) to not only control their blood glucose, but to stay alive.

TYPE 2 DIABETES

Type 2 diabetes is the most common form of diabetes. It is estimated that up to 90 percent of the people who have diabetes have type 2. The cause appears to be resistance to insulin's action compounded by a deficiency of insulin secretion.

People with type 2 diabetes are usually over age 35, are overweight, and have a family history of type 2 diabetes. Type 2 diabetes actually begins years before diagnosis, as an increasing resistance to insulin. This increasing resistance is the result of genetics, weight gain (especially abdominal fat), decreased activity, and aging. The major site of insulin resistance is the muscle tissue, which normally burns up the majority of the glucose in the bloodstream. When insulin has a difficult time "opening doors" on the body's cells, the pancreas tries to compensate by making more and more insulin. For some people, the pancreas is eventually unable to keep up with the increased workload. Blood glucose levels rise above normal after meals, and fasting glucose levels begin to remain above normal, too. Ironically, very high glucose levels can damage the beta cells, a condition called glucose toxicity. This further accelerates the breakdown of the pancreas' ability to control blood sugar levels. When glucose rises high enough to produce symptoms (excessive thirst, frequent urination, wounds that don't heal, for example), or when a complication such as a heart attack, stroke, visual disturbance, infection, numbness, or serious gum disease is treated, the diagnosis of type 2 diabetes is often made.

GESTATIONAL DIABETES

Gestational diabetes is diabetes that is diagnosed for the first time during pregnancy. It occurs in about 3 percent of all pregnancies. Gestational diabetes is diagnosed using a three-hour glucose tolerance test. If any two of the glucose readings during the test exceed the upper limits of normal, the diagnosis is made. Rarely are the glucose levels high enough to harm the mother. The problem is the mother's blood. Extra glucose flows to the developing baby, which then produces extra insulin. This, in turn, causes the baby to grow too quickly, resulting in a difficult labor and delivery.

Throughout the pregnancy, the mother's insulin resistance and glucose levels increase, right up to delivery. In 97 percent of cases, the mother's glucose levels

promptly return to normal after the baby and placenta are delivered. Many women with gestational diabetes can control their glucose levels during pregnancy through diet and exercise. Some, however, require insulin to keep glucose levels within a healthy range for the fetus.

Women who have had gestational diabetes have a significantly greater chance of developing diabetes later in life. Studies have shown that weight control and increased physical activity reduce the risk of future diabetes by as much as 50 percent.

YOUR DIABETES TOOL KIT

A well-stocked kit of tools helps you keep your blood sugar under tight control and ward off the frightening complications associated with diabetes.

MONITORING YOUR GLUCOSE

Blood glucose monitoring is a vital part of the diabetes management process, and frequent self-monitoring is a key to successful diabetes care. By checking your glucose, you get a precise measurement of what your blood glucose level is so you can adjust your food, medication, or activity level accordingly and with confidence. The blood glucose values are like clues in a mystery novel. The more clues you have, the greater your ability to solve the mystery. Of course, the opposite can be true as well. The less you check, the fewer clues you have and the more your diabetes remains a mystery to both you and your diabetes care team.

EATING FOR BETTER CONTROL

When you learned you had diabetes, you may have assumed you'd have to go on a special, restrictive diet. Perhaps you'd heard of people with diabetes who had to give up every food they enjoyed or who stopped going to certain events or restaurants because there was nothing they could eat there. Well, cheer up. You don't need to follow a "diabetic diet."

Your body needs adequate amounts of six essential nutrients to function normally. Three of these—water, vitamins, and minerals—provide no energy and do not affect blood glucose levels. The other three—carbohydrate, protein, and fat—provide your body with the energy it needs to work. This energy is measured in calories. Any food that contains calories can cause your blood glucose levels to rise. For your body to properly use these energy calories, it needs insulin. Whenever you eat, your food is digested and broken down or converted into your body's primary fuel source, glucose. While all energy nutrients are broken down into glucose, carbohydrates have a more direct effect on blood glucose levels. Protein and fat have a slower, more indirect effect on those levels. Understanding this can help you predict how food will affect your glucose levels.

To be successful in diabetes self-care, you need to make personal food choices that are compatible with your blood glucose goals and your tastes. Since carbohydrates have the greatest direct effect on glucose levels, determining the amount of carbohydrates that your body can manage well is a cornerstone in your glucose management.

The first step is for you to eat absolutely normally. Have the foods you usually eat, in the amounts you normally have, as frequently as you usually have them. Check food labels to determine which foods contain carbohydrate, then keep a running tally of the total grams of carbohydrate you eat throughout the entire day. Take detailed, honest notes.

Along with taking these notes, you need to test your blood glucose levels. Testing allows you to see how well your insulin level matches your carbohydrate intake. No matter its source, insulin works with the food you eat. If you eat too much food for the insulin that is available, your glucose level will be too high; if you eat too little, your glucose level will be too low.

Eating a variety of foods will also help ensure that you get the nutrients you need—not just the carbohydrate, protein, and fat but also the vitamins and minerals that are essential to good health.

STAYING ACTIVE

Activity is one of the three cornerstones in the treatment of diabetes, along with food and medication. Moving toward a more physically active life is generally inexpensive, convenient, easy, and usually produces great rewards in terms of blood glucose control (due to improved insulin sensitivity) and a general feeling of well-being.

USING MEDICATIONS TO TREAT DIABETES

For many people who have type 2 diabetes, using food and activity to control blood glucose is not enough. For them, diabetes medications can be lifesavers—helping to lower blood glucose levels and stave off diabetes complications.

People with type 1 diabetes make very little, if any, insulin, so they are dependent on insulin injections. Insulin injections have become extremely safe and simple, and virtually pain-free. And, they remain the most natural and effective way to treat high blood sugar in these individuals.

On the other hand, individuals with type 2 diabetes may depend on pills to help lower blood glucose levels. But there are usually multiple problems that need to be addressed, and one pill just can't do it all. Problems include insulin resistance by the body's cells, oversecretion of glucose by the liver, insufficient insulin production by the pancreas, and alternated rates of food digestion. Sometimes a combination of medications is much more effective at lowering glucose levels than is a single medicine.

WEIGHING THE BENEFITS

You may realize (or your doctor has told you) that being overweight—especially carrying too much fat in your abdominal area—hampers diabetes control. For people with diabetes, the best path to weight loss is the same one that leads to getting well and staying well. There's no denying weight loss is beneficial for people with type 2 diabetes who are overweight. Even a weight loss of just 5 to 10 percent of your total body weight can bring impressive improvements to your health. Studies show that when a person who has recently been diagnosed with diabetes loses weight, blood glucose levels drop, blood pressure improves, and cholesterol levels return to a healthier range. Medications may be decreased or even stopped altogether.

TAKING COMMAND OF YOUR CARE

The right approach to diabetes treatment puts YOU in charge. Not your doctor. Not your spouse. YOU. You become the boss of your diabetes team, choosing the staff that best serves your needs, tracking your progress, and

keeping your eyes on the ultimate goal— your health and well-being.

YOUR DIABETES TEAM

Surround yourself with knowledgeable, trustworthy, and expert advisors— your diabetes care team—who can help you get the information, advice, treatments, and support you need to manage your diabetes effectively. This team should include your doctor (possibly an endocrinologist who typically has the most experience and skill in diabetes care) and a registered dietitian nutritionist (RDN) who may also be certified as a diabetes educator (CDE) to teach people with diabetes how to manage the disease. Also onboard should be a pharmacist, dentist, mental-health professional, eye doctor, podiatrist, and cardiologist, as needed.

Your team will help you choose what, how much, and when to eat; help you become more physically active; assist with your medications; check your blood glucose; and teach you all they can about diabetes.

YOU'RE ON YOUR WAY

Once you feel comfortable with your meal and activity plan, checking your blood sugar, and managing your medication, you'll be able to enjoy the great taste of food without worries. Use the following recipes to get started on the path to a healthier lifestyle.

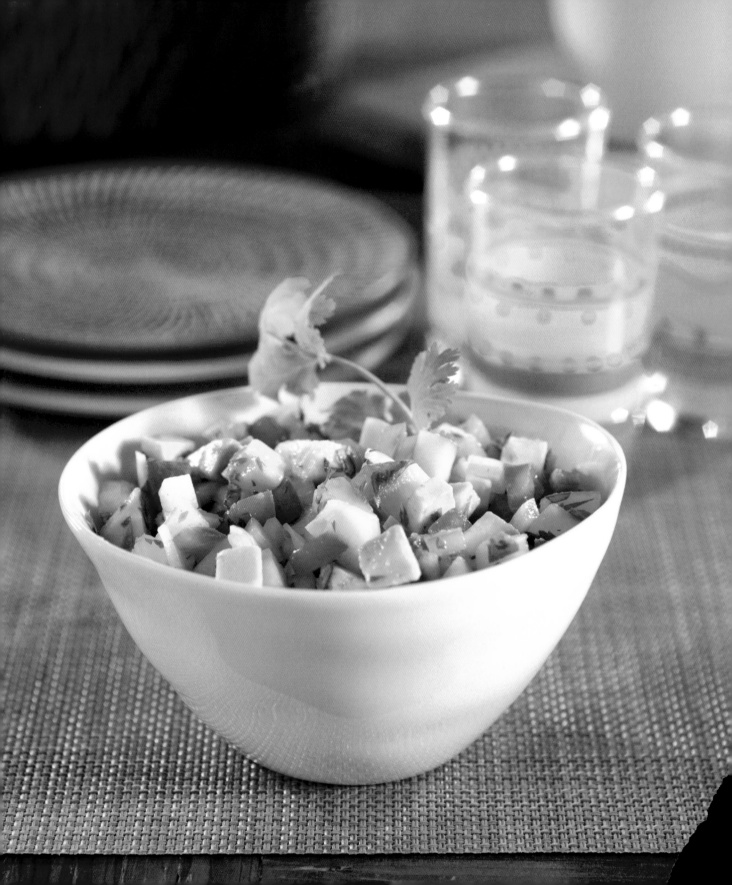

APPETIZERS & STARTERS

AVOCADO SALSA

MAKES 32 SERVINGS (ABOUT 4 CUPS)

1 medium avocado, diced

1 cup chopped onion

1 cup chopped peeled cucumber

1 Anaheim or jalapeño pepper,* seeded and chopped

½ cup chopped fresh tomato

2 tablespoons chopped fresh cilantro, plus additional for garnish

½ teaspoon salt

¼ teaspoon hot pepper sauce

Peppers can sting and irritate the skin, so wear rubber gloves when handling peppers and do not touch your eyes.

1. Combine avocado, onion, cucumber, Anaheim pepper, tomato, 2 tablespoons cilantro, salt and hot pepper sauce in medium bowl; mix gently.

2. Cover and refrigerate at least 1 hour before serving. Garnish with additional cilantro.

PER SERVING

CALORIES
13

TOTAL FAT
1g

SATURATED FAT
1g

CHOLESTEROL
0mg

SODIUM
38mg

CARBS
1g

DIETARY FIBER
1g

PROTEIN
1g

DIETARY EXCHANGES

free

SHRIMP AND WATERMELON CEVICHE

MAKES 28 SERVINGS

- 1 **pound medium raw shrimp, peeled and deveined**
- ½ **cup plus 2 tablespoons lime juice, divided**
- 1 **cup finely chopped seedless watermelon**
- ½ **cup finely chopped jicama**
- ½ **cup finely chopped red onion**
- ½ **cup chopped fresh cilantro**
- 1 **jalapeño pepper,* minced**
- 56 **water crackers**

*Jalapeño peppers can sting and irritate the skin, so wear rubber gloves when handling peppers and do not touch your eyes.

1. Chop shrimp into small pieces. Combine shrimp and ½ cup lime juice in medium bowl; toss gently. Cover and refrigerate 1 hour or until shrimp are pink and opaque. Drain and discard liquid.

2. Combine watermelon, jicama, onion, cilantro, jalapeño pepper and remaining 2 tablespoons lime juice in large bowl; mix well. Gently stir in shrimp. Cover and refrigerate at least 30 minutes to allow flavors to blend.

3. Serve with crackers.

Note
The shrimp aren't traditionally cooked; the citric acid from the lime juice "cooks" the shrimp while they are marinating.

PER SERVING

CALORIES
44

TOTAL FAT
1g

SATURATED FAT
0g

CHOLESTEROL
20mg

SODIUM
132mg

CARBS
7g

DIETARY FIBER
1g

PROTEIN
3g

DIETARY EXCHANGES

½ bread/starch

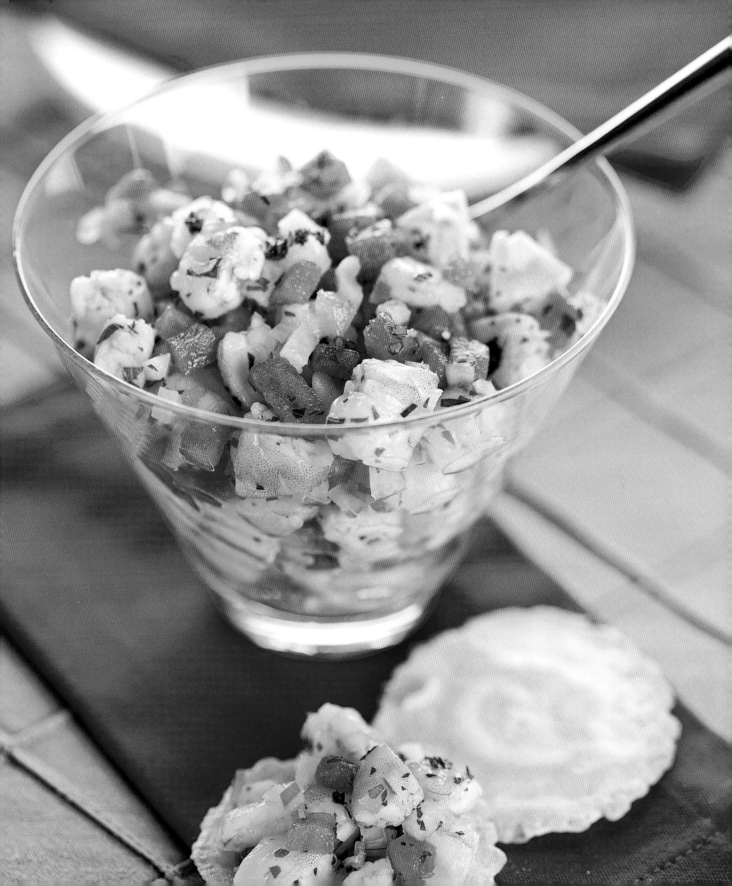

BUFFALO CAULIFLOWER BITES

MAKES 8 SERVINGS

- ¾ cup all-purpose flour
- ¼ cup cornstarch
- ½ teaspoon garlic powder
- ½ teaspoon black pepper
- 1 cup water
- 1 large head cauliflower (2½ pounds), cut into 1-inch florets
- ½ cup hot pepper sauce
- ¼ cup (½ stick) butter, melted
- Celery sticks, blue cheese or ranch dressing (optional)

1. Preheat oven to 450°F. Line sheet pan with foil; spray with nonstick cooking spray.

2. Whisk flour, cornstarch, garlic powder and black pepper in large bowl. Whisk in water until smooth and well blended. Add cauliflower to batter in batches; stir to coat. Arrange on prepared sheet pan.

3. Bake 20 minutes or until cauliflower is lightly browned. Combine hot pepper sauce and butter in small bowl; mix well. Pour over cauliflower; toss until well blended. Bake 5 to 10 minutes or until cauliflower is glazed and crisp, stirring as necessary. Serve with celery sticks and dressing, if desired.

PER SERVING

CALORIES
150

TOTAL FAT
6g

SATURATED FAT
4g

CHOLESTEROL
15mg

SODIUM
550mg

CARBS
20g

DIETARY FIBER
3g

PROTEIN
4g

DIETARY EXCHANGES

½ bread/starch, 1½ vegetable, 1 fat

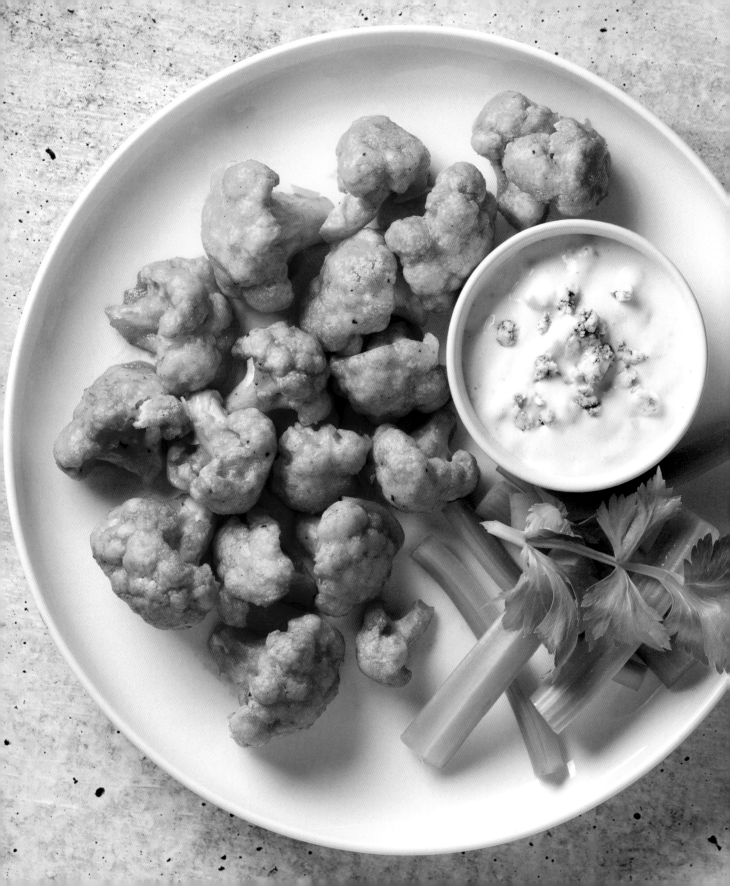

SAVORY PUMPKIN HUMMUS

MAKES 12 SERVINGS (ABOUT 1½ CUPS)

1 can (15 ounces) solid-pack pumpkin

3 tablespoons chopped fresh parsley, plus additional for garnish

3 tablespoons tahini

3 tablespoons lemon juice

3 cloves garlic

1 teaspoon ground cumin

½ teaspoon salt

⅛ teaspoon black pepper

⅛ teaspoon ground red pepper, plus additional for garnish

Assorted vegetable sticks

1. Combine pumpkin, 3 tablespoons parsley, tahini, lemon juice, garlic, cumin, salt, black pepper and ⅛ teaspoon ground red pepper in food processor or blender; process until smooth. Cover and refrigerate at least 2 hours to allow flavors to develop.

2. Sprinkle with additional ground red pepper, if desired. Garnish with additional parsley. Serve with assorted vegetable sticks.

PER SERVING

CALORIES
38

TOTAL FAT
2g

SATURATED FAT
0g

CHOLESTEROL
0mg

SODIUM
101mg

CARBS
4g

DIETARY FIBER
1g

PROTEIN
1g

DIETARY EXCHANGES

1 vegetable, ½ fat

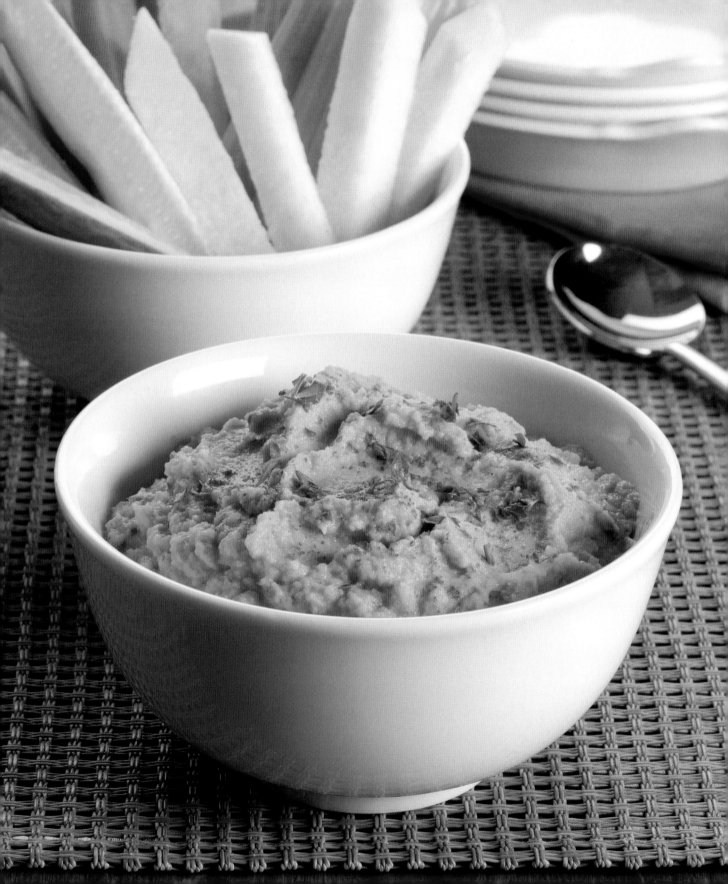

SMOKED SALMON SPIRALS

MAKES 2 SERVINGS (3 SLICES EACH)

- 2 tablespoons low-fat cream cheese
- 1 light sun-dried tomato flatbread
- 2 ounces smoked salmon (lox)
- ½ cup baby arugula
- ½ cup thinly sliced red bell pepper

Spread cream cheese on flatbread. Layer with smoked salmon, arugula and bell pepper. Roll up jelly-roll style. To serve, cut into 6 pieces.

PER SERVING

CALORIES
121

TOTAL FAT
5g

SATURATED FAT
2g

CHOLESTEROL
15mg

SODIUM
800mg

CARBS
12g

DIETARY FIBER
5g

PROTEIN
11g

DIETARY EXCHANGES

1 bread/starch, 1 meat

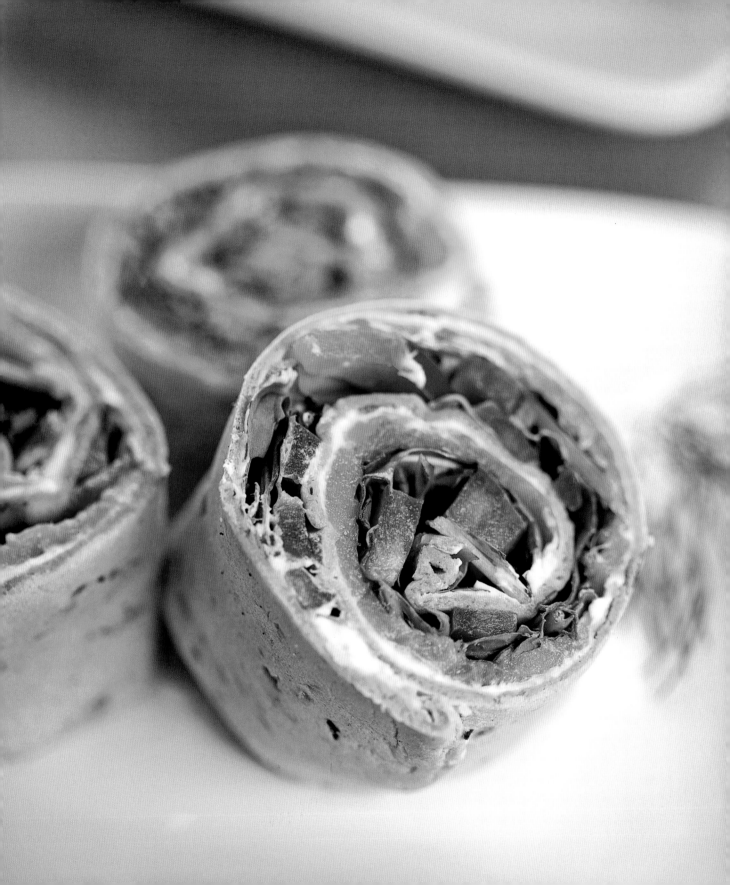

MINI MARINATED BEEF SKEWERS

MAKES 6 SERVINGS (3 SKEWERS EACH)

1 boneless beef top round steak (about 1 pound)

2 tablespoons reduced-sodium soy sauce

1 tablespoon dry sherry

1 teaspoon dark sesame oil

2 cloves garlic, minced

18 fresh greens and cherry tomatoes (optional)

1. Cut beef crosswise into 18 (⅛-inch-thick) slices. Place in large resealable food storage bag. Add soy sauce, sherry, oil and garlic. Seal bag; turn to coat. Marinate in refrigerator at least 30 minutes or up to 2 hours.

2. Meanwhile, soak 18 (6-inch) wooden skewers in water 20 minutes.

3. Preheat broiler. Drain beef; discard marinade. Weave beef accordion-style onto skewers. Place on rack of broiler pan.

4. Broil 4 to 5 inches from heat 2 minutes. Turn skewers over; broil 2 minutes more or until beef is barely pink. Serve warm with greens and tomatoes, if desired.

PER SERVING

CALORIES
120

TOTAL FAT
4g

SATURATED FAT
1g

CHOLESTEROL
60mg

SODIUM
99mg

CARBS
2g

DIETARY FIBER
1g

PROTEIN
20g

DIETARY EXCHANGES

2 meat

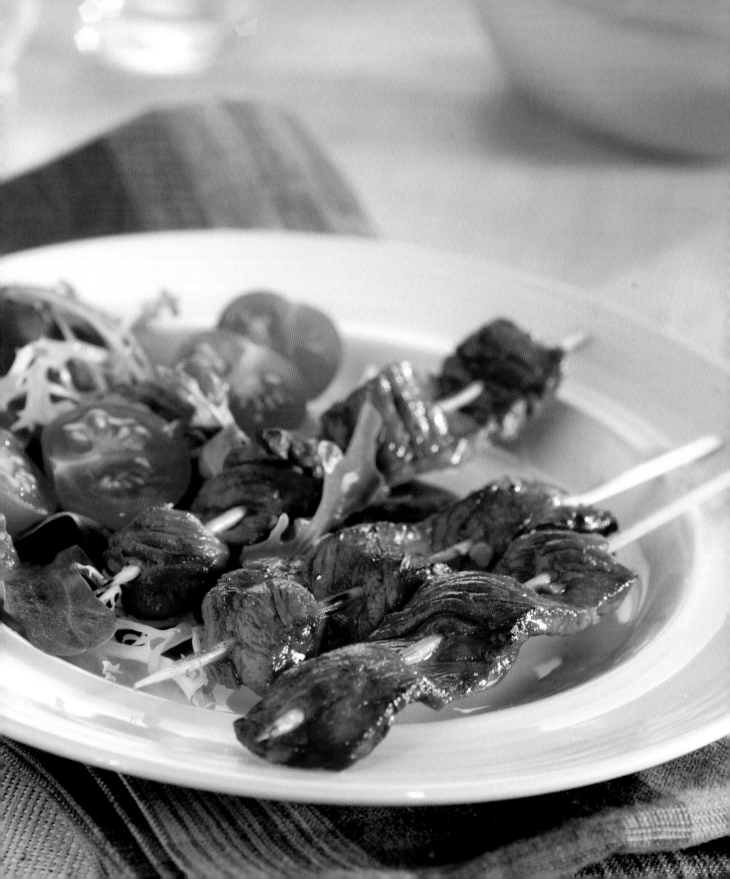

ASIAN VEGETABLE ROLLS WITH SOY-LIME DIPPING SAUCE

MAKES 6 SERVINGS (3 ROLLS EACH)

¼ cup reduced-sodium soy sauce

2 tablespoons lime juice

1 clove garlic, crushed

1 teaspoon honey

½ teaspoon finely chopped fresh ginger

¼ teaspoon dark sesame oil

⅛ to ¼ teaspoon red pepper flakes

½ cup grated cucumber

⅓ cup grated carrot

¼ cup sliced yellow bell pepper (1 inch long)

2 tablespoons thinly sliced green onion

18 small lettuce leaves

Sesame seeds (optional)

1. Combine soy sauce, lime juice, garlic, honey, ginger, oil and red pepper flakes in small bowl.

2. Combine cucumber, carrot, bell pepper and green onion in medium bowl. Stir in 1 tablespoon soy sauce mixture.

3. Place about 1 tablespoon vegetable mixture on each lettuce leaf. Roll up leaves; sprinkle with sesame seeds, if desired. Serve with remaining sauce for dipping.

PER SERVING

CALORIES
25

TOTAL FAT
1g

SATURATED FAT
1g

CHOLESTEROL
0mg

SODIUM
343mg

CARBS
5g

DIETARY FIBER
1g

PROTEIN
1g

DIETARY EXCHANGES

free

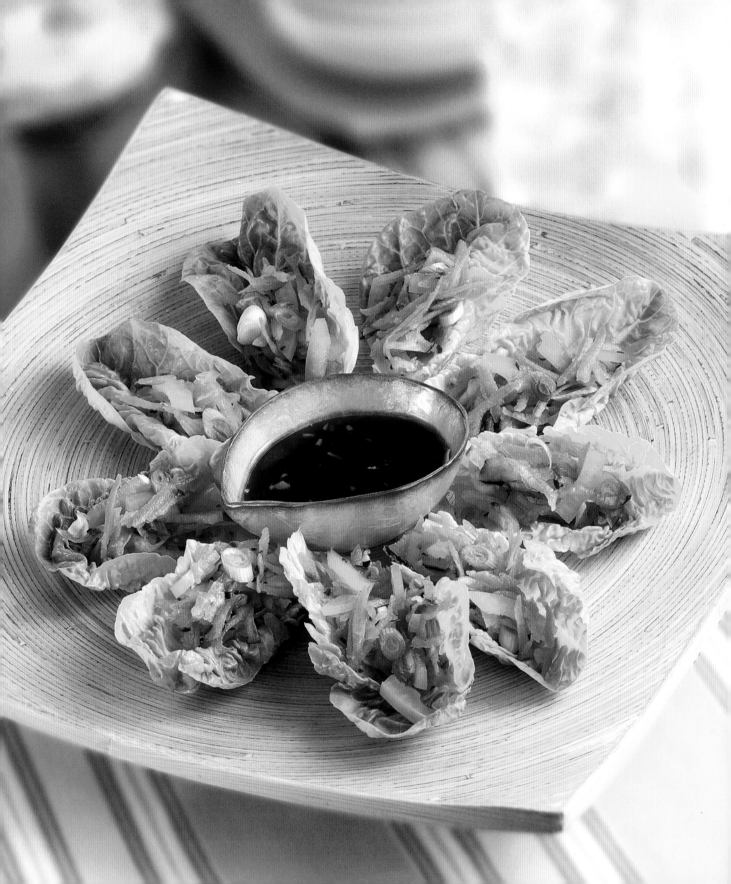

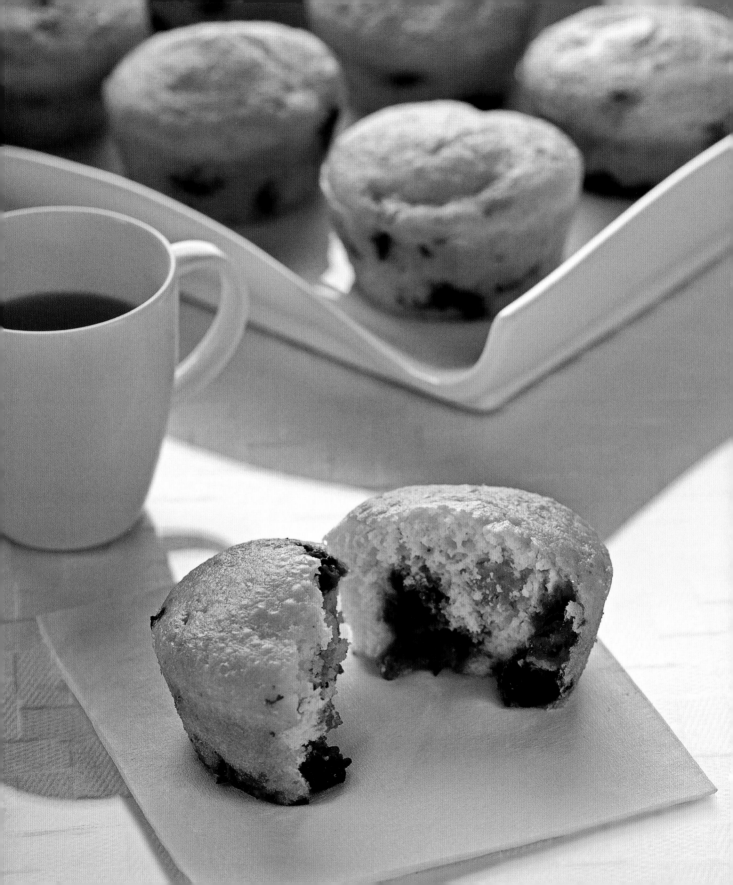

START OFF YOUR DAY

SWEET & SAVORY BREAKFAST MUFFINS

MAKES 12 MUFFINS

1¼ cups original pancake and baking mix

1 cup fat-free (skim) milk

3 egg whites

¼ cup maple syrup

4 small fully cooked turkey breakfast sausage links, diced

1 cup fresh blueberries

1. Preheat oven to 375°F. Spray 12 standard (2½-inch) muffin cups with nonstick cooking spray.

2. Stir pancake mix, milk, egg whites and maple syrup in large bowl until smooth and well blended. Fold in sausage and blueberries. Pour evenly into prepared muffin cups.

3. Bake 18 to 20 minutes or until toothpick inserted into centers comes out clean. Serve warm.

PER SERVING

CALORIES
80

TOTAL FAT
1g

SATURATED FAT
0g

CHOLESTEROL
5mg

SODIUM
310mg

CARBS
14g

DIETARY FIBER
1g

PROTEIN
4g

DIETARY EXCHANGES

1 bread/starch

BANANA-PECAN BREAD

MAKES 1 LOAF (ABOUT 16 SERVINGS)

- 3 large ripe bananas, mashed (about 1⅓ cups)
- ½ cup packed dark brown sugar
- ¼ cup granulated sugar
- 2 eggs, lightly beaten
- ¼ cup fat-free (skim) milk
- ¼ cup canola oil
- 2 cups reduced-fat biscuit baking mix
- 1 teaspoon ground cinnamon
- ½ cup golden raisins
- ½ cup chopped pecans

1. Preheat oven to 350°F. Spray 9×5-inch loaf pan with nonstick cooking spray; dust with flour.

2. Combine bananas, brown sugar, granulated sugar, eggs, milk and oil in large bowl; mix well. Stir in baking mix and cinnamon until well blended. Fold in raisins and pecans. Pour batter into prepared pan.

3. Bake 45 to 50 minutes or until top is golden brown and toothpick inserted into center comes out clean. Cool in pan on wire rack 20 minutes. Remove to wire rack; serve warm or cool completely.

PER SERVING

CALORIES
183

TOTAL FAT
8g

SATURATED FAT
1g

CHOLESTEROL
23mg

SODIUM
176mg

CARBS
28g

DIETARY FIBER
1g

PROTEIN
3g

DIETARY EXCHANGES

2 bread/starch, 1 fat

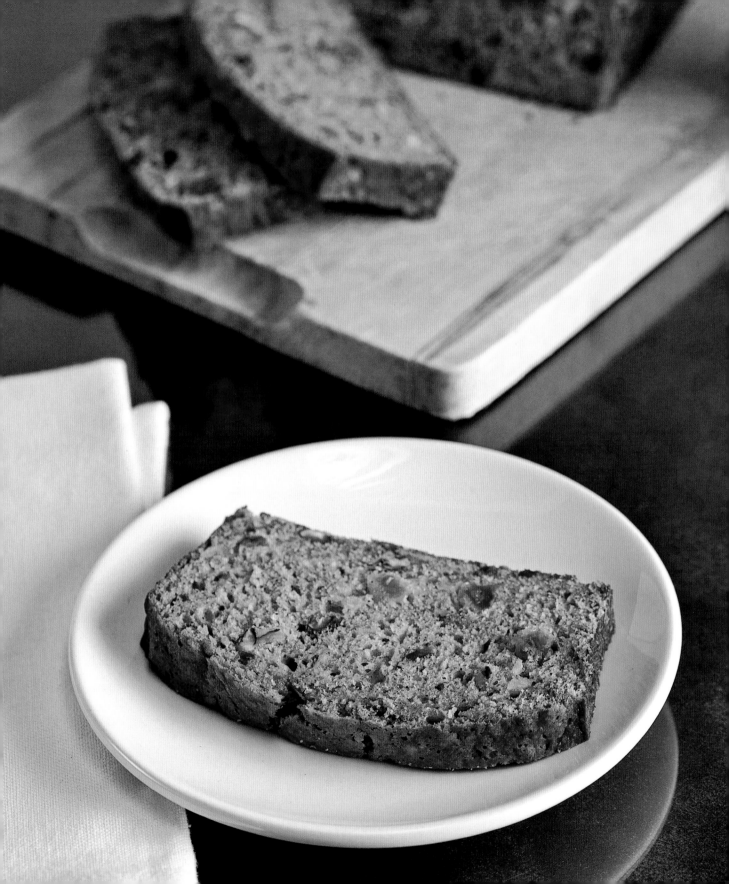

GERMAN APPLE PANCAKE

MAKES 6 SERVINGS

1 tablespoon butter

1 large *or* 2 small apples, peeled and thinly sliced (about 1½ cups)

1 tablespoon packed brown sugar

1½ teaspoons ground cinnamon, divided

2 eggs

2 egg whites

1 tablespoon granulated sugar

1 teaspoon vanilla

¼ teaspoon salt

½ cup all-purpose flour

½ cup milk

Maple syrup (optional)

1. Preheat oven to 425°F.

2. Melt butter in medium cast iron or ovenproof skillet* over medium heat. Add apples, brown sugar and ½ teaspoon cinnamon; cook and stir 5 minutes or until apples just begin to soften. Remove from heat. Arrange apple slices in single layer in skillet.

3. Whisk eggs, egg whites, granulated sugar, remaining 1 teaspoon cinnamon, vanilla and salt in medium bowl until well blended. Stir in flour and milk until smooth and well blended. Pour evenly over apples.

4. Bake 20 to 25 minutes or until puffed and golden brown. Serve with maple syrup, if desired.

To make skillet ovenproof, wrap handle in foil.

Note

Pancake will fall slightly after being removed from the oven.

PER SERVING

CALORIES
120

TOTAL FAT
2.5g

SATURATED FAT
0.5g

CHOLESTEROL
75mg

SODIUM
160mg

CARBS
18g

DIETARY FIBER
1g

PROTEIN
5g

DIETARY EXCHANGES

1 bread/starch, ½ fat

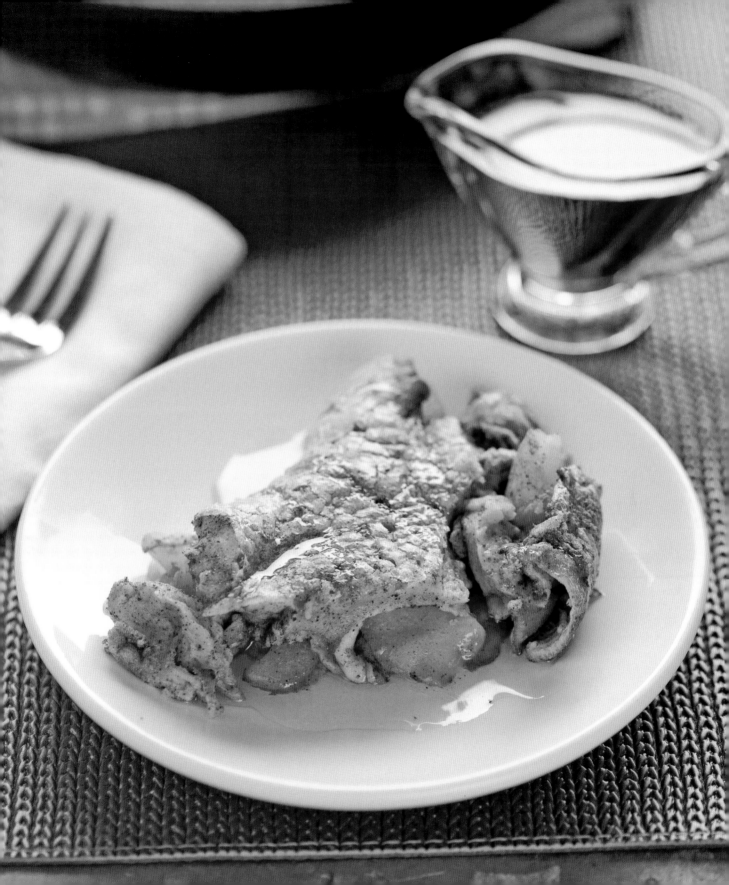

HARVEST APPLE OATMUG

MAKES 1 SERVING

1 cup water

½ cup old-fashioned oats

½ cup chopped Granny Smith apple

2 tablespoons raisins

1 teaspoon packed brown sugar

¼ teaspoon ground cinnamon

⅛ teaspoon salt

Microwave Directions

1. Combine water, oats, apple, raisins, brown sugar, cinnamon and salt in large microwavable mug; mix well.

2. Microwave on HIGH 1½ minutes; stir. Microwave on HIGH 1 minute or until thickened and liquid is absorbed. Let stand 1 to 2 minutes before serving.

PER SERVING

CALORIES
251

TOTAL FAT
3g

SATURATED FAT
1g

CHOLESTEROL
0mg

SODIUM
302mg

CARBS
54g

DIETARY FIBER
6g

PROTEIN
6g

DIETARY EXCHANGES

2 bread/starch, 1½ fruit

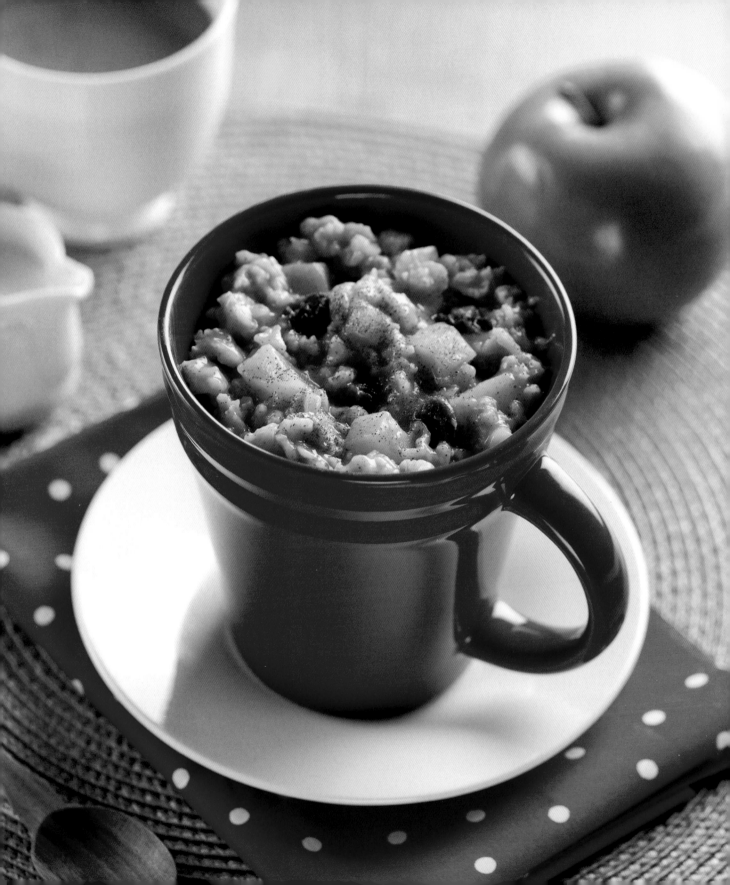

BREAKFAST PIZZA MARGHERITA

MAKES 6 SERVINGS

1 (12-inch) prepared pizza crust

3 slices 95% fat-free turkey bacon

2 cups cholesterol-free egg substitute

½ cup fat-free (skim) milk

1½ tablespoons chopped fresh basil, divided

⅛ teaspoon black pepper

2 plum tomatoes, thinly sliced

½ cup (2 ounces) shredded reduced-fat mozzarella cheese

¼ cup (1 ounce) shredded reduced-fat Cheddar cheese

1. Preheat oven to 450°F. Place pizza crust on 12-inch pizza pan. Bake 6 to 8 minutes or until heated through.

2. Meanwhile, coat large skillet with nonstick cooking spray. Cook bacon over medium-high heat until crisp. Remove from skillet to paper towels; cool. Crumble bacon.

3. Combine egg substitute, milk, ½ tablespoon basil and pepper in medium bowl. Coat same skillet with cooking spray. Add egg substitute mixture. Cook over medium heat until mixture begins to set around edges. Gently stir eggs, allowing uncooked portions to flow underneath. Repeat stirring of egg mixture every 1 to 2 minutes or until eggs are just set. Remove from heat.

4. Arrange tomato slices on warmed pizza crust. Spoon scrambled eggs over tomatoes. Sprinkle with bacon. Top with cheeses. Bake 1 minute or until cheeses are melted. Sprinkle with remaining 1 tablespoon basil. Cut into 6 wedges. Serve immediately.

PER SERVING

CALORIES
311

TOTAL FAT
9g

SATURATED FAT
2g

CHOLESTEROL
11mg

SODIUM
675mg

CARBS
35g

DIETARY FIBER
2g

PROTEIN
21g

DIETARY EXCHANGES

2 bread/starch,
2 meat,
½ vegetable,
1½ fat

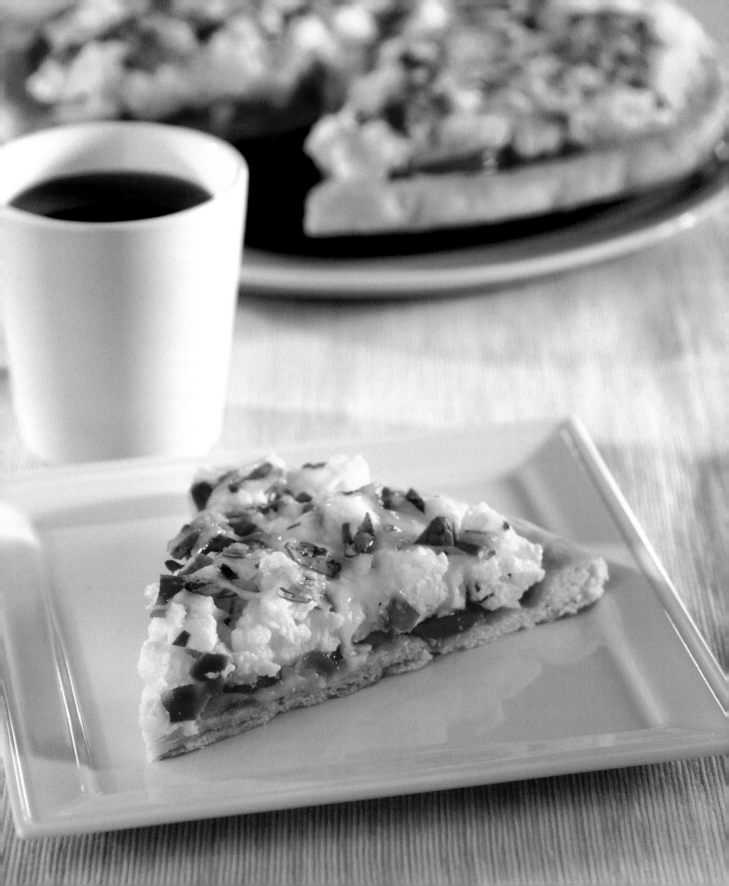

PB BANANA MUFFINS

MAKES 18 MUFFINS

¾ cup all-purpose flour

¾ cup whole wheat flour

1 teaspoon baking soda

½ teaspoon salt

¾ cup reduced-fat creamy peanut butter

2 ripe bananas, mashed (about 1 cup)

½ cup packed brown sugar

½ cup plain nonfat yogurt

1 egg

¼ cup honey

¼ cup vegetable oil

1 teaspoon vanilla

1. Preheat oven to 375°F. Line 18 standard (2½-inch) muffin cups with paper baking cups or spray with nonstick cooking spray.

2. Combine all-purpose flour, whole wheat flour, baking soda and salt in medium bowl; mix well. Beat peanut butter, bananas, brown sugar, yogurt, egg, honey, oil and vanilla in large bowl with electric mixer at medium speed until smooth and well blended. Add flour mixture; beat on low speed just until combined. Spoon batter evenly into prepared muffin cups.

3. Bake 15 to 18 minutes or until toothpick inserted into centers comes out clean. Cool in pans 5 minutes. Remove to wire racks; cool completely.

PER SERVING

CALORIES
184

TOTAL FAT
8g

SATURATED FAT
1g

CHOLESTEROL
10mg

SODIUM
223mg

CARBS
25g

DIETARY FIBER
2g

PROTEIN
4g

DIETARY EXCHANGES

1½ bread/starch, 1½ fat

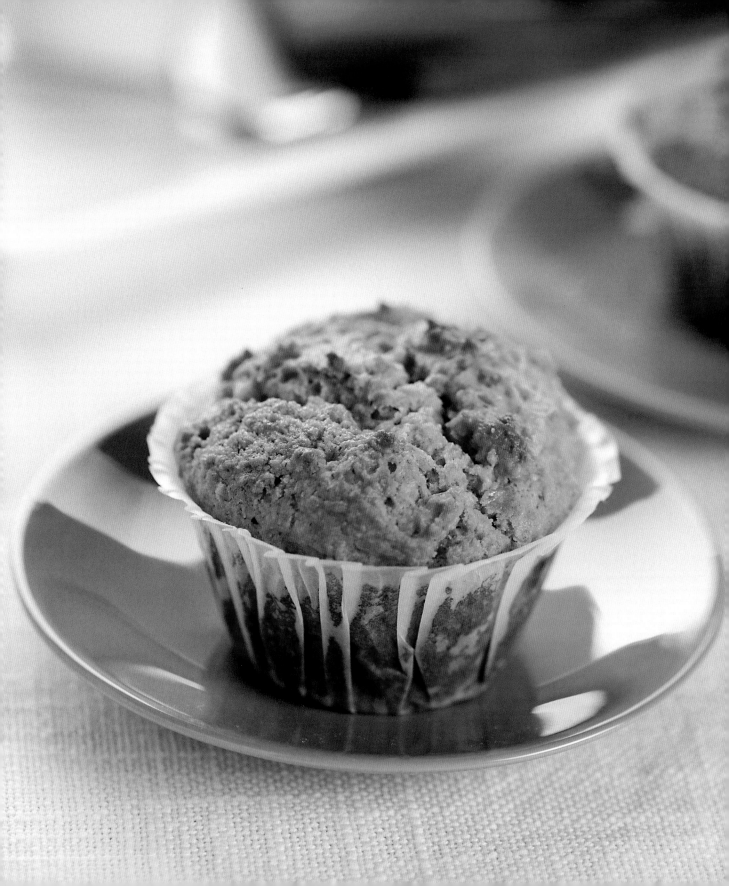

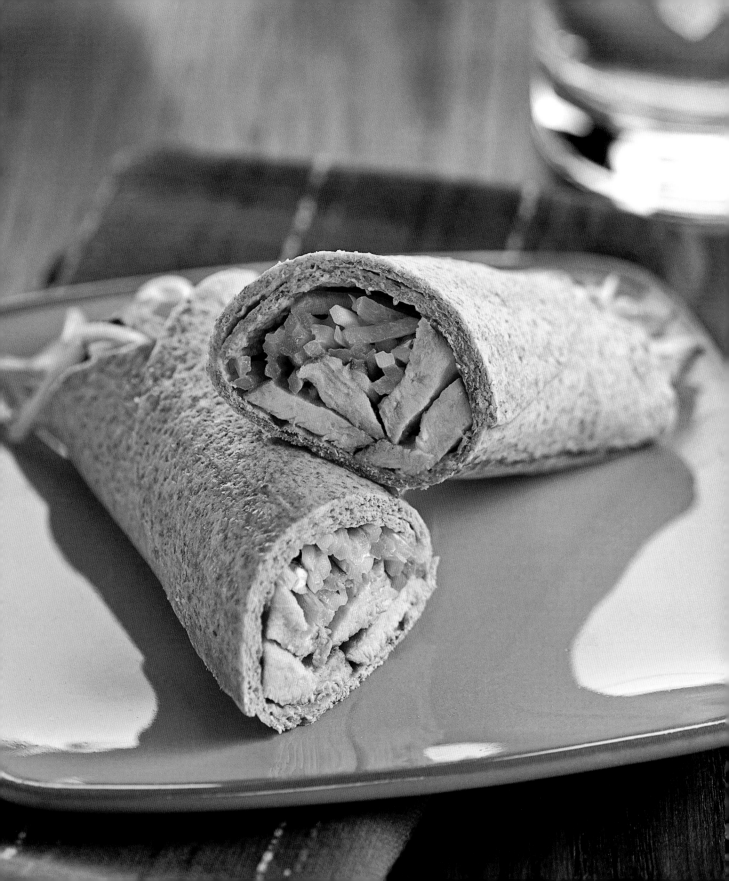

LUNCH & LIGHTER BITES

GRILLED BUFFALO CHICKEN WRAPS

MAKES 4 SERVINGS

4 boneless skinless chicken breasts (about 4 ounces each)

¼ cup plus 2 tablespoons buffalo wing sauce, divided

2 cups broccoli slaw

1 tablespoon light blue cheese salad dressing

4 (8-inch) whole wheat tortillas, warmed

1. Place chicken in large resealable food storage bag. Add ¼ cup buffalo sauce; seal bag. Marinate in refrigerator 15 minutes.

2. Meanwhile, prepare grill for direct cooking over medium-high heat. Grill chicken 5 to 6 minutes per side or until no longer pink. When cool enough to handle, slice chicken and combine with remaining 2 tablespoons buffalo sauce in medium bowl.

3. Combine broccoli slaw and blue cheese dressing in medium bowl; mix well.

4. Arrange chicken and broccoli slaw evenly down center of each tortilla. Roll up to secure filling. To serve, cut in half diagonally.

Tip

If you don't like the spicy flavor of buffalo wing sauce, substitute your favorite barbecue sauce.

PER SERVING

CALORIES
290

TOTAL FAT
8g

SATURATED FAT
2g

CHOLESTEROL
65mg

SODIUM
790mg

CARBS
25g

DIETARY FIBER
5g

PROTEIN
28g

DIETARY EXCHANGES

1 bread/starch,
1 meat,
1 vegetable, ½ fat

THAI CHICKEN PIZZA

MAKES 6 SERVINGS

- 1 **package (10 ounces) ready-made whole wheat pizza crust**
- ¼ **cup peanut sauce**
- ⅓ **cup chopped fresh cilantro, plus additional for garnish**
- 1¼ **cups (4 ounces) shredded cooked chicken**
- ½ **cup diced cucumber**
- ¾ **cup fresh or canned bean sprouts, rinsed and drained**
- ¾ **cup shredded or matchstick carrots**
- ⅓ **cup sliced green onions**

1. Preheat oven to 450°F. Place pizza crust on baking sheet. Spread peanut sauce in thin layer over crust within ½ inch of edge. Sprinkle with ⅓ cup cilantro. Arrange chicken evenly over crust. Bake 8 minutes or until warm.

2. Sprinkle cucumber, bean sprouts, carrots and green onions over top of pizza. Cut into squares or wedges and garnish with additional cilantro.

PER SERVING

CALORIES
220

TOTAL FAT
5g

SATURATED FAT
2g

CHOLESTEROL
22mg

SODIUM
418mg

CARBS
30g

DIETARY FIBER
6g

PROTEIN
15g

DIETARY EXCHANGES

2 bread/starch, 1 meat

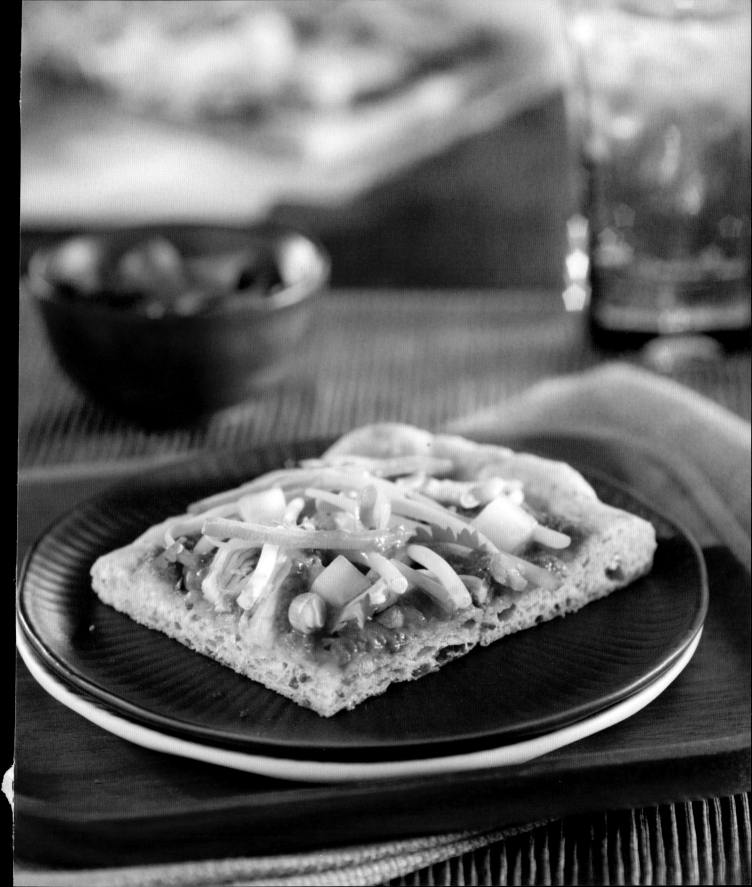

LENTIL BURGERS

MAKES 4 SERVINGS

- 1 can (about 14 ounces) vegetable broth
- 1 cup dried lentils, rinsed and sorted
- 1 small carrot, grated
- ¼ cup coarsely chopped mushrooms
- 1 egg
- ¼ cup plain dry bread crumbs
- 3 tablespoons finely chopped onion
- 2 to 4 cloves garlic, minced
- 1 teaspoon dried thyme
- ¼ cup plain fat-free yogurt
- ¼ cup chopped seeded cucumber
- ½ teaspoon dried mint
- ¼ teaspoon dried dill weed
- ¼ teaspoon black pepper
- ⅛ teaspoon salt

  Dash hot pepper sauce (optional)

  Kaiser rolls (optional)

1. Bring broth to a boil in medium saucepan over high heat. Stir in lentils; reduce heat to low. Simmer, covered, about 30 minutes or until lentils are tender and liquid is absorbed. Cool to room temperature.

2. Place lentils, carrot and mushrooms in food processor or blender; process until finely chopped but not smooth. (Some whole lentils should still be visible.) Stir in egg, bread crumbs, onion, garlic and thyme. Refrigerate, covered, 2 to 3 hours.

3. Shape lentil mixture into 4 (½-inch-thick) patties. Spray large skillet with nonstick cooking spray; heat over medium heat. Cook patties over medium-low heat about 10 minutes or until browned on both sides.

4. Meanwhile, for sauce, combine yogurt, cucumber, mint, dill weed, black pepper, salt and hot pepper sauce, if desired, in small bowl. Serve burgers on rolls with sauce.

PER SERVING

CALORIES
124

TOTAL FAT
2g

SATURATED FAT
1g

CHOLESTEROL
54mg

SODIUM
166mg

CARBS
21g

DIETARY FIBER
1g

PROTEIN
9g

DIETARY EXCHANGES

½ bread/starch,
½ meat,
2½ vegetable

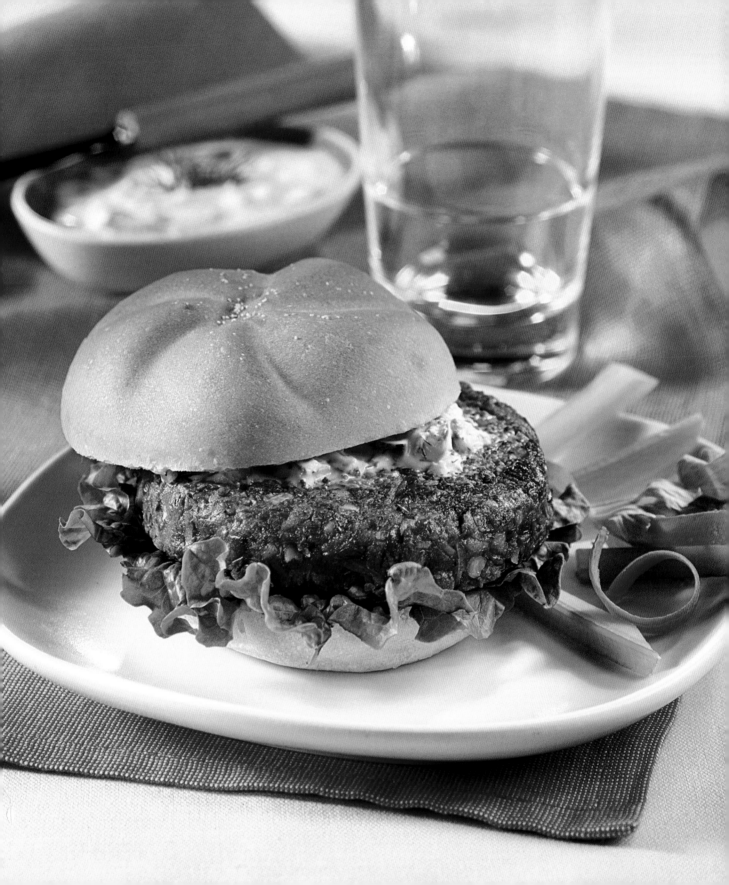

PEPPER PITA PIZZAS

MAKES 4 SERVINGS

1 teaspoon olive oil

1 medium onion, thinly sliced

1 medium red bell pepper, cut into thin strips

1 medium green bell pepper, cut into thin strips

4 cloves garlic, minced

2 tablespoons minced fresh basil *or* 2 teaspoons dried basil

1 tablespoon minced fresh oregano *or* 1 teaspoon dried oregano

2 Italian plum tomatoes, coarsely chopped

4 (6-inch) pita bread rounds

1 cup (4 ounces) shredded reduced-fat Monterey Jack cheese

1. Preheat oven to 425°F. Heat oil in medium nonstick skillet over medium heat until hot. Add onion, bell peppers, garlic, basil and oregano. Partially cover; cook 5 minutes or until tender, stirring occasionally. Add tomatoes. Partially cover and cook 3 minutes.

2. Place pita rounds on baking sheet. Divide tomato mixture evenly among pitas; top each pita with ¼ cup cheese. Bake 5 minutes or until cheese is melted.

PER SERVING

CALORIES
302

TOTAL FAT
7g

SATURATED FAT
3g

CHOLESTEROL
20mg

SODIUM
552mg

CARBS
44g

DIETARY FIBER
2g

PROTEIN
16g

DIETARY EXCHANGES

2 bread/starch, 1½ meat, 2½ vegetable, ½ fat

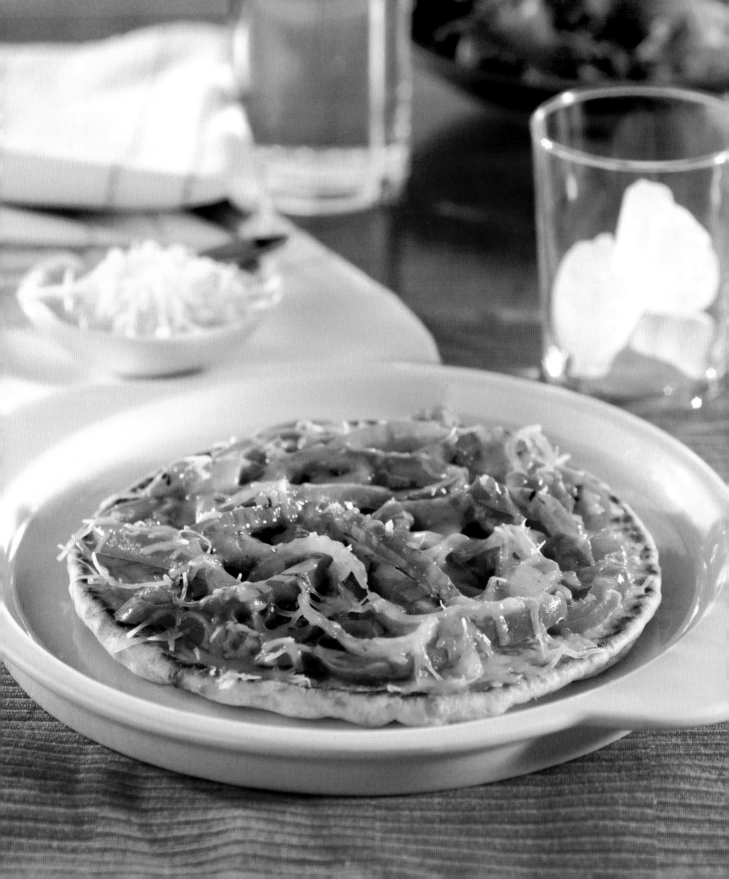

SHRIMP CAPRESE PASTA

MAKES 4 SERVINGS

1 cup uncooked whole wheat penne

2 teaspoons olive oil

2 cups coarsely chopped grape tomatoes

4 tablespoons chopped fresh basil, divided

1 tablespoon balsamic vinegar

2 cloves garlic, minced

¼ teaspoon salt

⅛ teaspoon red pepper flakes

8 ounces medium raw shrimp, peeled and deveined (with tails on)

1 cup grape tomatoes, halved

2 ounces fresh mozzarella pearls

1. Cook pasta according to package directions, omitting salt. Drain, reserving ½ cup cooking water. Set aside.

2. Heat oil in large skillet over medium heat. Add 2 cups chopped tomatoes, reserved ½ cup pasta water, 2 tablespoons basil, vinegar, garlic, salt and red pepper flakes. Cook and stir 10 minutes or until tomatoes begin to soften.

3. Add shrimp and 1 cup halved tomatoes to skillet; cook and stir 5 minutes or until shrimp turn pink and opaque. Add pasta; cook until heated through.

4. Divide mixture evenly among 4 bowls. Top evenly with cheese and remaining 2 tablespoons basil.

PER SERVING

CALORIES
222

TOTAL FAT
6g

SATURATED FAT
2g

CHOLESTEROL
81mg

SODIUM
550mg

CARBS
27g

DIETARY FIBER
4g

PROTEIN
17g

DIETARY EXCHANGES

1½ bread/starch, 1½ meat, 1 vegetable

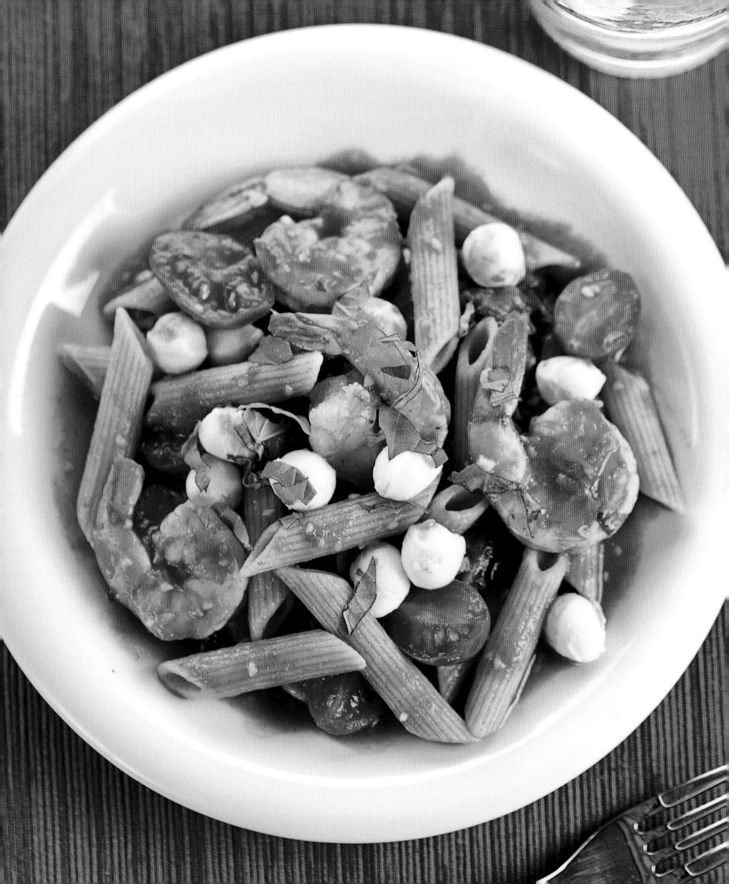

GRILLED STEAK AND BLUE CHEESE FLATBREADS

MAKES 2 SERVINGS

- 1 (4-ounce) filet mignon
- ¼ teaspoon garlic powder
- ⅛ teaspoon salt
- ⅛ teaspoon black pepper
- 2 light blue cheese spreadable cheese wedges (about 1 ounce each)
- 2 light original flatbreads
- ½ cup thinly sliced tomato
- ¼ cup thinly sliced red onion
- 2 tablespoons crumbled reduced-fat blue cheese
- ½ cup baby arugula
  Balsamic vinegar (optional)

1. Prepare grill for direct cooking over medium heat.

2. Season filet with garlic powder, salt and pepper. Grill 5 minutes per side or until medium rare or desired doneness. Remove to plate. Let stand 5 minutes. Reduce heat to low.

3. Slice filet into thin slices. Spread 1 cheese wedge onto each flatbread. Top evenly with filet slices, tomato and onion. Sprinkle with blue cheese.

4. Grill, covered, 8 to 10 minutes or until crisp and heated through. Top with arugula just before serving. Drizzle with balsamic vinegar, if desired.

PER SERVING

CALORIES
127

TOTAL FAT
5g

SATURATED FAT
2g

CHOLESTEROL
19mg

SODIUM
357mg

CARBS
10g

DIETARY FIBER
5g

PROTEIN
13g

DIETARY EXCHANGES

½ bread/starch, 1½ meat, ½ vegetable

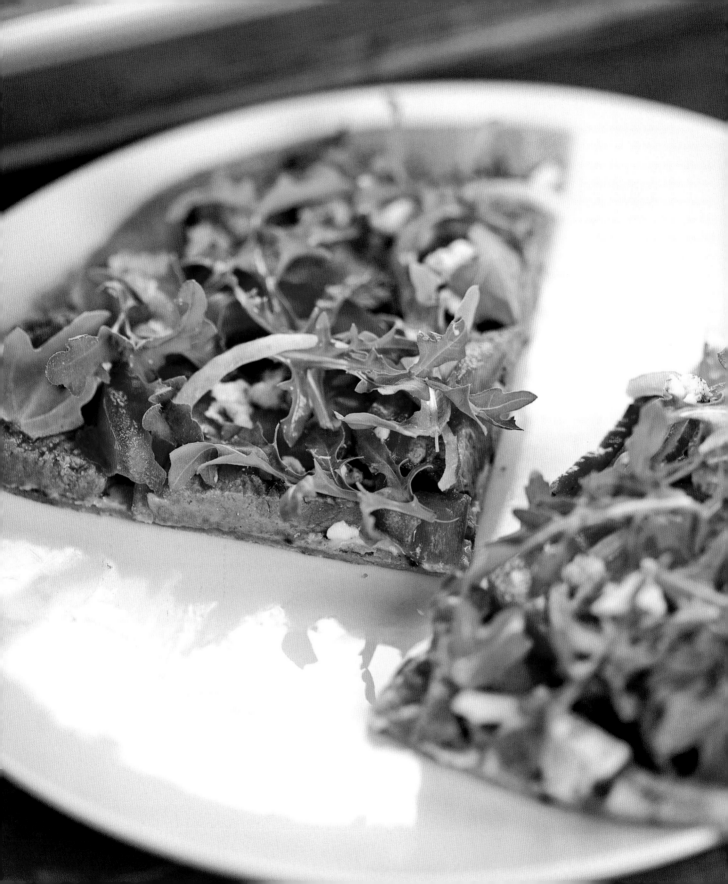

PESTO TUNA MELTS

MAKES 2 SERVINGS

- 1 **can (5 ounces) tuna in water, drained and flaked**
- 1 **tablespoon plain nonfat Greek yogurt**
- 1 **tablespoon pesto sauce**
- 1 **teaspoon lemon juice**
- ⅛ **teaspoon black pepper**
- 2 **light multi-grain English muffins, split**
- 4 **tomato slices**
- 6 **teaspoons shredded reduced-fat mozzarella cheese**

1. Preheat oven to 350°F.

2. Combine tuna, yogurt, pesto, lemon juice and pepper in small bowl; gently mix.

3. Divide tuna mixture evenly among English muffin halves. Top each half with 1 tomato slice and 1½ teaspoons cheese.

4. Bake 8 to 10 minutes or until cheese is melted.

PER SERVING

CALORIES
270

TOTAL FAT
6g

SATURATED FAT
1g

CHOLESTEROL
30mg

SODIUM
580mg

CARBS
32g

DIETARY FIBER
1g

PROTEIN
21g

DIETARY EXCHANGES

2 bread/starch, 2 meat, 1 fat

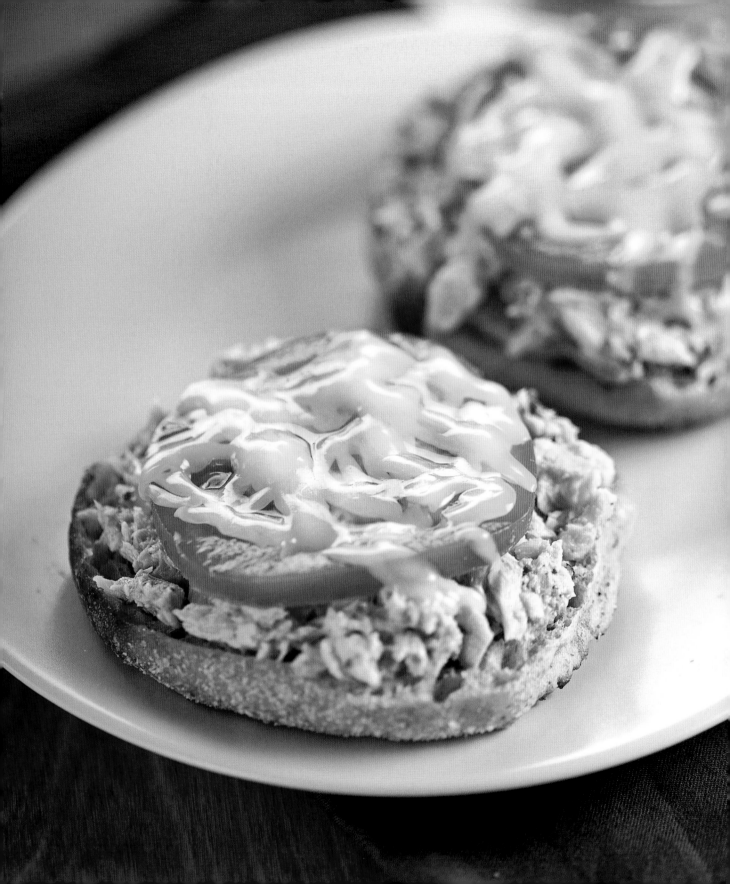

SUMMER'S BOUNTY PASTA WITH BROCCOLI PESTO

MAKES 4 SERVINGS

- 2 cups broccoli florets
- 2 cups uncooked bowtie (farfalle) pasta
- ½ cup loosely packed fresh basil leaves
- 5 tablespoons shredded Parmesan-Romano cheese blend, divided
- 2 tablespoons chopped walnuts, toasted*
- 1½ tablespoons extra virgin olive oil
- 2 cloves garlic, crushed, divided
- ⅛ teaspoon salt
- 6 ounces medium cooked shrimp
- ¼ teaspoon black pepper
- 1 package (6 ounces) fresh baby spinach
- 1 cup halved grape tomatoes

To toast walnuts, cook in small skillet over medium heat 1 to 2 minutes or lightly browned, stirring frequently.

1. Bring large saucepan of water to a boil. Add broccoli; cook 3 minutes or until tender. Remove to small bowl with slotted spoon; reserve water.

2. Cook pasta according to package directions using reserved water, omitting salt. Drain pasta; cover to keep warm.

3. Combine broccoli, basil, 3 tablespoons cheese, walnuts, oil, 1 clove garlic and salt in food processor or blender; process until smooth. Stir into pasta in saucepan; toss to coat. Cover to keep warm.

4. Spray large skillet with nonstick cooking spray; heat over medium heat. Add shrimp, remaining 1 clove garlic and pepper; cook and stir until heated through. Stir in spinach and tomatoes; cook until spinach is wilted and tomatoes begin to soften. Add to pasta; stir gently to combine.

5. Divide pasta mixture evenly among 4 serving bowls; top with remaining 2 tablespoons cheese.

PER SERVING

CALORIES
263

TOTAL FAT
12g

SATURATED FAT
3g

CHOLESTEROL
94mg

SODIUM
638mg

CARBS
22g

DIETARY FIBER
4g

PROTEIN
20g

DIETARY EXCHANGES

1 bread/starch,
2 meat,
2 vegetable,
½ fat

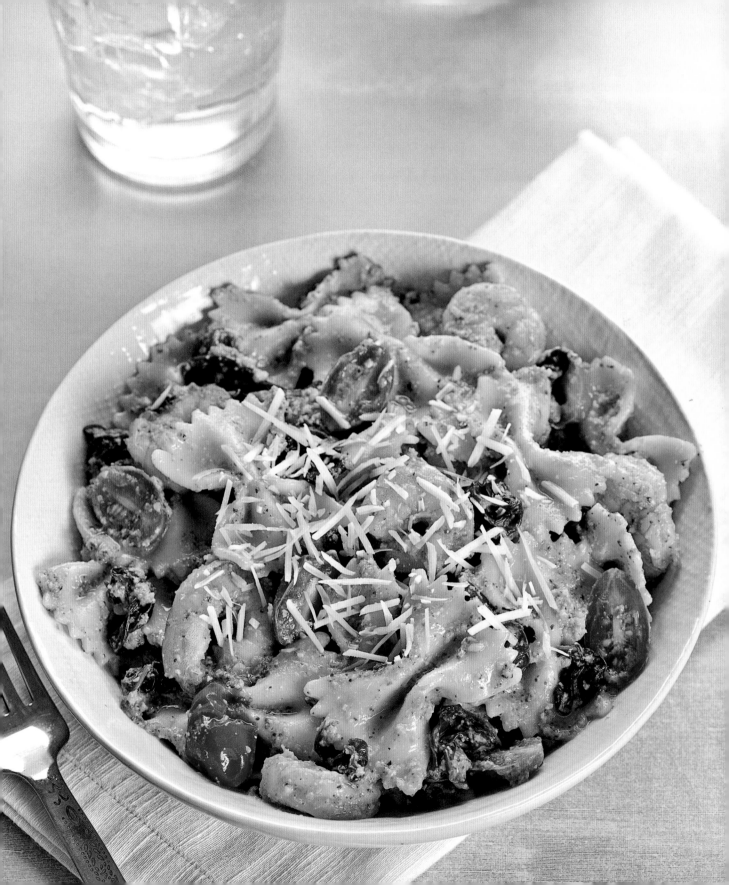

QUINOA BURRITO BOWLS

MAKES 4 SERVINGS

1 cup uncooked quinoa

2 cups water

2 tablespoons fresh lime juice, divided

¼ cup light sour cream

2 teaspoons vegetable oil

1 small onion, diced

1 red bell pepper, diced

1 clove garlic, minced

½ cup canned black beans, rinsed and drained

½ cup thawed frozen corn

Shredded lettuce

Lime wedges (optional)

1. Place quinoa in fine-mesh strainer; rinse well under cold running water. Bring 2 cups water to a boil in small saucepan; stir in quinoa. Reduce heat to low; cover and simmer 10 to 15 minutes or until quinoa is tender and water is absorbed. Stir in 1 tablespoon lime juice. Cover and keep warm. Combine sour cream and remaining 1 tablespoon lime juice in small bowl; set aside.

2. Meanwhile, heat oil in large skillet over medium heat. Add onion and bell pepper; cook and stir 5 minutes or until softened. Add garlic; cook 1 minute. Add black beans and corn; cook 3 to 5 minutes or until heated through.

3. Divide quinoa among 4 serving bowls; top with black bean mixture, lettuce and sour cream mixture. Garnish with lime wedges.

PER SERVING

CALORIES
258

TOTAL FAT
7g

SATURATED FAT
1g

CHOLESTEROL
4mg

SODIUM
136mg

CARBS
42g

DIETARY FIBER
6g

PROTEIN
9g

DIETARY EXCHANGES

3 bread/starch, 1 fat

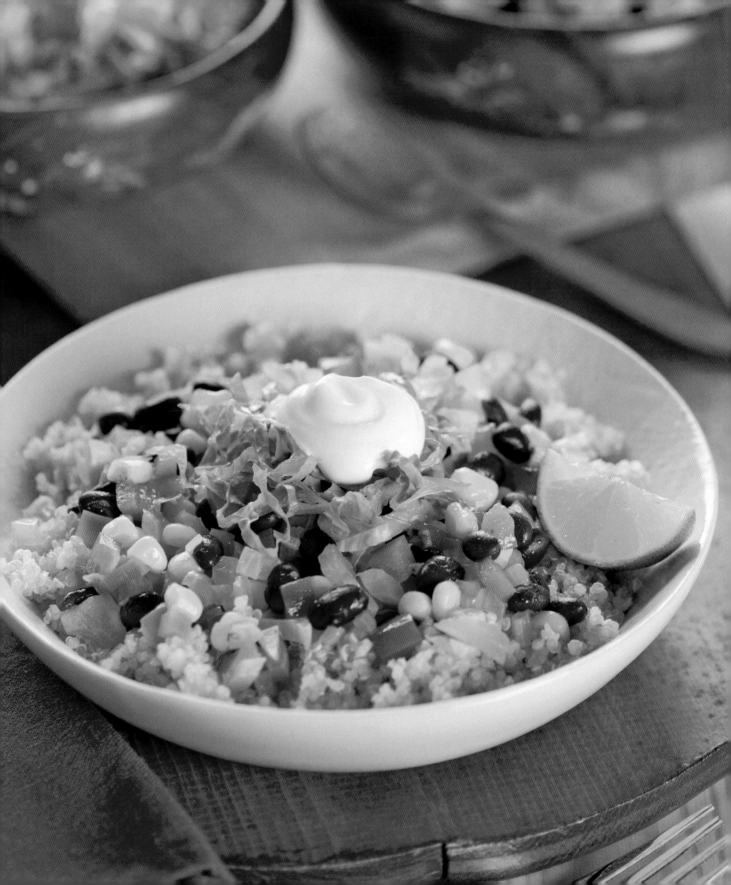

ROASTED EGGPLANT PANINI

MAKES 4 SANDWICHES

1 medium eggplant
(about 1¼ pounds)

1 cup (4 ounces)
shredded reduced-
fat mozzarella
cheese

1 tablespoon chopped
fresh basil

1 tablespoon fresh
lemon juice

⅛ teaspoon salt

8 slices (1 ounce each)
whole grain Italian
bread

1. Preheat oven to 400°F. Line baking sheet with parchment paper; spray with nonstick cooking spray. Slice eggplant in half lengthwise. Place cut sides down on prepared baking sheet. Roast 45 minutes. Let stand 15 minutes or until cool enough to handle.

2. Meanwhile, combine cheese, basil, lemon juice and salt in small bowl; set aside.

3. Cut each eggplant piece in half. Remove pulp; discard skin. Place one fourth of eggplant on each of 4 bread slices, pressing gently into bread. Top evenly with cheese mixture. Top with remaining bread slices. Spray sandwiches with nonstick cooking spray.

4. Heat large nonstick grill pan or skillet over medium heat. Cook sandwiches 3 to 4 minutes per side, pressing down with spatula until cheese is melted and bread is toasted. (Cover pan during last minute of cooking to melt cheese, if desired.) Serve immediately.

PER SERVING

CALORIES
310

TOTAL FAT
7g

SATURATED FAT
2g

CHOLESTEROL
10mg

SODIUM
275mg

CARBS
50g

DIETARY FIBER
9g

PROTEIN
19g

DIETARY EXCHANGES

3 bread/starch,
2 meat

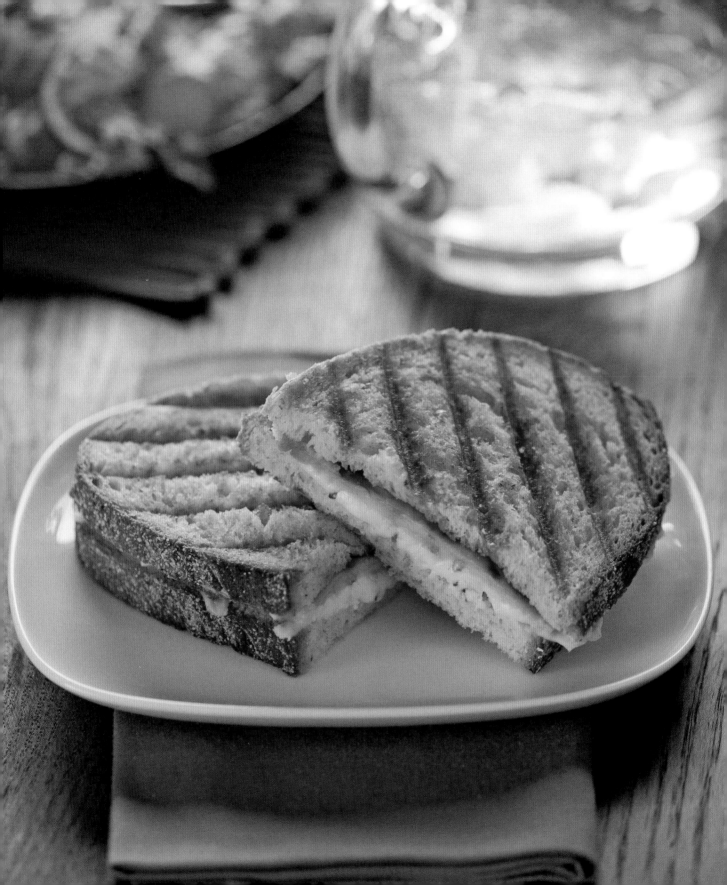

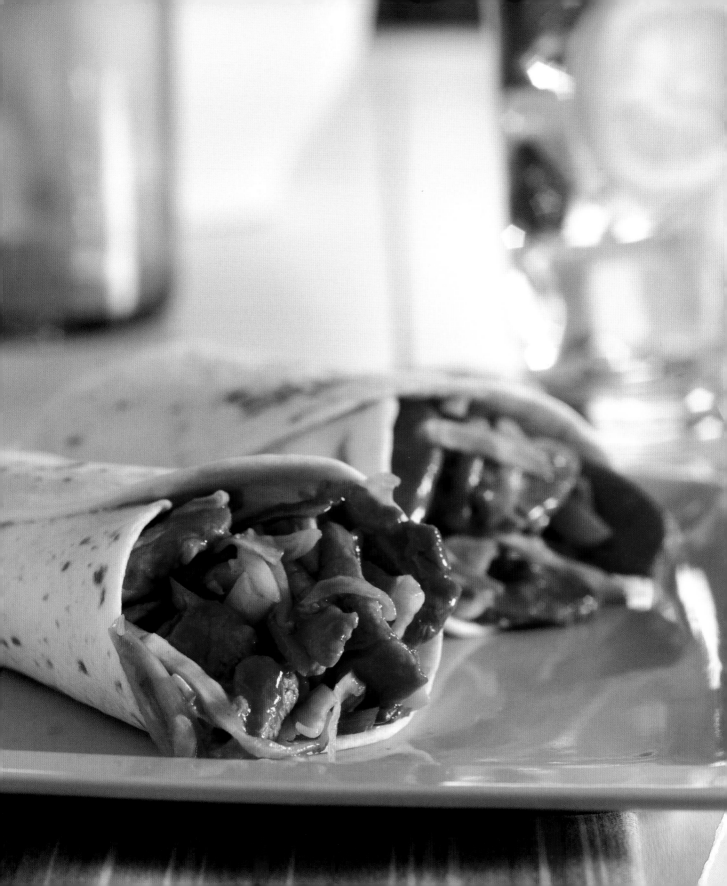

DINNERTIME FIXES

EASY MOO SHU PORK

MAKES 2 SERVINGS

- 7 ounces pork tenderloin, sliced
- 4 green onions, cut into ½-inch pieces
- 1½ cups packaged coleslaw mix
- 2 tablespoons hoisin sauce or Asian plum sauce
- 4 (8-inch) fat-free flour tortillas, warmed

1. Spray large nonstick skillet with nonstick cooking spray; heat over medium-high heat. Add pork and green onions; stir-fry 2 to 3 minutes or until pork is barely pink in center. Stir in coleslaw mix and hoisin sauce.

2. Spoon pork mixture onto tortillas. Roll up tortillas, folding in sides to enclose filling.

Note
To warm tortillas, stack and wrap loosely in plastic wrap. Microwave on HIGH 15 to 20 seconds or until hot and pliable.

PER SERVING

CALORIES
293

TOTAL FAT
4g

SATURATED FAT
1g

CHOLESTEROL
58mg

SODIUM
672mg

CARBS
37g

DIETARY FIBER
14g

PROTEIN
26g

DIETARY EXCHANGES
2 bread/starch,
2 meat,
1 vegetable

GREEK CHICKEN BURGERS WITH CUCUMBER YOGURT SAUCE

MAKES 4 SERVINGS

½ cup plus 2 tablespoons plain nonfat Greek yogurt

½ medium cucumber, peeled, seeded and finely chopped

Juice of ½ lemon

3 cloves garlic, minced, divided

2 teaspoons finely chopped fresh mint *or* ½ teaspoon dried mint

⅛ teaspoon salt

⅛ teaspoon ground white pepper

1 pound ground chicken breast

¾ cup (3 ounces) crumbled reduced-fat feta cheese

4 large kalamata olives, rinsed, patted dry and minced

1 egg

½ to 1 teaspoon dried oregano

¼ teaspoon black pepper

Mixed baby lettuce (optional)

Fresh mint leaves (optional)

1. Combine yogurt, cucumber, lemon juice, 2 cloves garlic, 2 teaspoons chopped mint, salt and white pepper in medium bowl; mix well. Cover and refrigerate until ready to serve.

2. Combine chicken, feta cheese, olives, egg, oregano, black pepper and remaining 1 clove garlic in large bowl; mix well. Shape mixture into 4 patties.

3. Spray grill pan with nonstick cooking spray; heat over medium-high heat. Grill patties 5 to 7 minutes per side or until cooked through (165°F).

4. Serve burgers with sauce and mixed greens, if desired. Garnish with mint leaves.

PER SERVING

CALORIES
260

TOTAL FAT
14g

SATURATED FAT
5g

CHOLESTEROL
150mg

SODIUM
500mg

CARBS
4g

DIETARY FIBER
1g

PROTEIN
29g

DIETARY EXCHANGES

3 meat,
½ vegetable,
1 fat

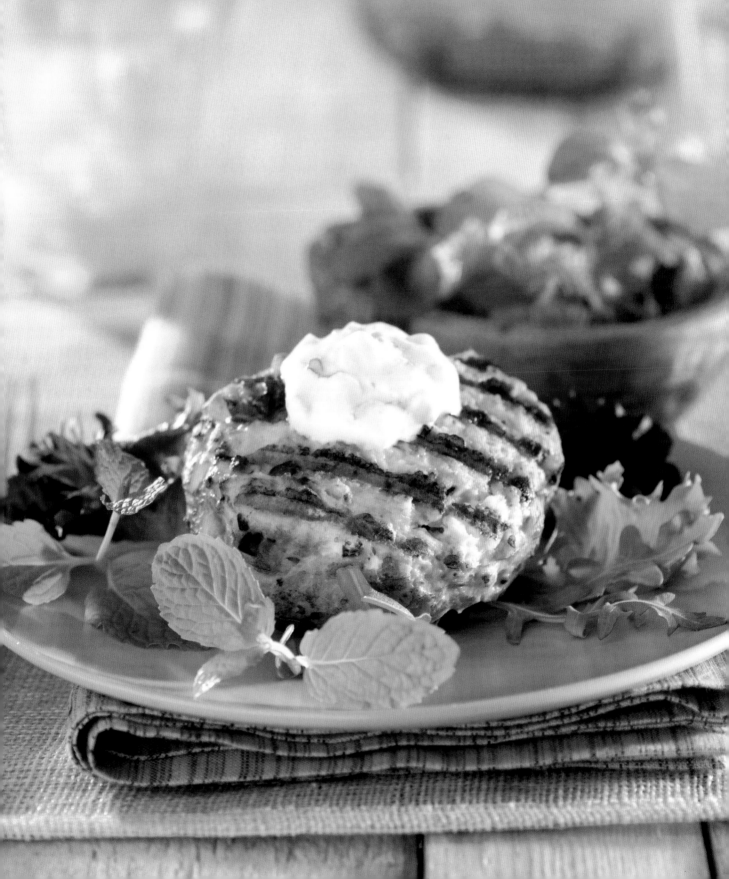

WHOLE WHEAT PENNE WITH BROCCOLI AND SAUSAGE

MAKES 6 SERVINGS

- 6 **to 7 ounces uncooked whole wheat penne pasta**
- 8 **ounces broccoli florets**
- 8 **ounces mild Italian turkey sausage, casings removed**
- 1 **medium onion, quartered and sliced**
- 2 **cloves garlic, minced**
- 2 **teaspoons grated lemon peel**
- ¼ **teaspoon salt**
- ⅛ **teaspoon black pepper**
- ⅓ **cup grated Parmesan cheese**

1. Cook pasta according to package directions, omitting salt. Add broccoli during last 5 to 6 minutes of cooking. Drain well; cover and keep warm.

2. Meanwhile, heat large nonstick skillet over medium heat. Crumble sausage into skillet. Add onion; cook until sausage is brown, stirring to break up meat. Drain fat. Add garlic; cook and stir 1 minute.

3. Add sausage mixture, lemon peel, salt and pepper to pasta mixture; toss until blended. Sprinkle Parmesan cheese evenly over each serving.

PER SERVING

CALORIES
208

TOTAL FAT
6g

SATURATED FAT
1g

CHOLESTEROL
26mg

SODIUM
425mg

CARBS
26g

DIETARY FIBER
4g

PROTEIN
13g

DIETARY EXCHANGES

1½ bread/starch,
2 meat,
1 vegetable, 1 fat

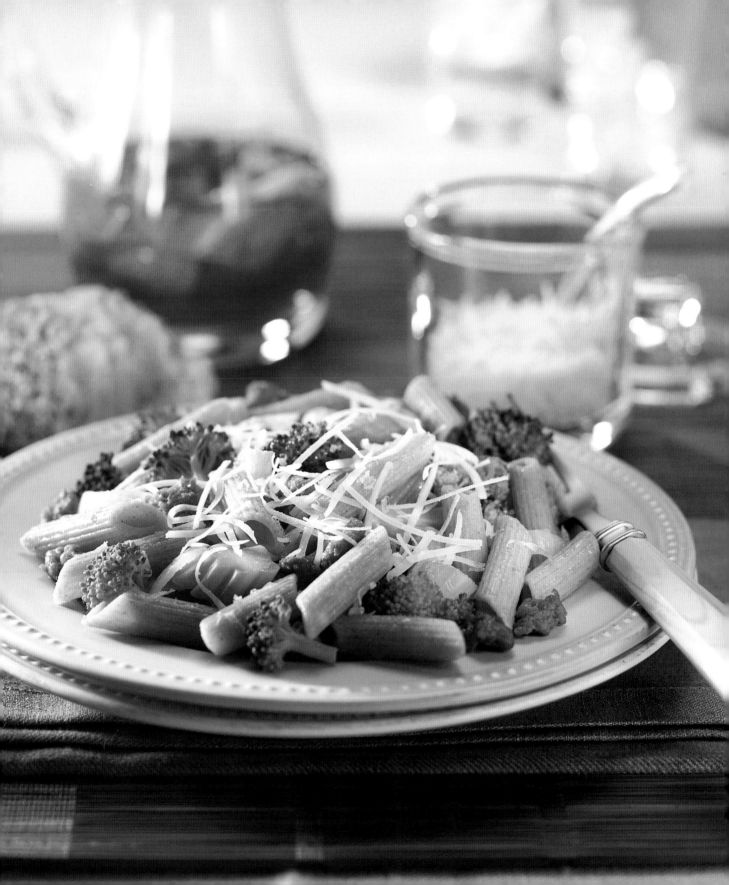

SPICY GINGER CHICKEN AND RICE TOSS

MAKES 4 SERVINGS

- 1 package (10 ounces) frozen brown rice
- 2 tablespoons canola oil
- 1 medium red onion, diced
- 1 medium red bell pepper, cut into 2-inch strips
- 4 medium cloves garlic, minced
- 1 tablespoon grated fresh ginger
- ⅛ to ¼ teaspoon red pepper flakes
- ¾ teaspoon salt
- 1½ cups diced cooked chicken breast (about 8 ounces)
- 1½ cups fresh or frozen thawed shelled edamame
- ½ cup chopped fresh cilantro
- 1 ounce slivered almonds, toasted*

*To toast almonds, spread in small skillet. Cook over medium heat 1 to 2 minutes or until nuts are lightly browned, stirring frequently.

1. Cook rice according to package directions.

2. Meanwhile, heat oil in large nonstick skillet over medium-high heat. Add onion and bell pepper; cook and stir 5 minutes or until onion begins to brown. Stir in garlic, ginger, red pepper flakes and salt; cook and stir 30 seconds. Add chicken and edamame; cook and stir 2 minutes or until heated through.

3. Remove from heat; stir in rice and cilantro. Let stand 5 minutes for flavors to blend. Sprinkle with almonds.

PER SERVING

CALORIES
326

TOTAL FAT
12g

SATURATED FAT
1g

CHOLESTEROL
40mg

SODIUM
476mg

CARBS
30g

DIETARY FIBER
7g

PROTEIN
26g

DIETARY EXCHANGES

2 bread/starch,
3 meat,
½ fat

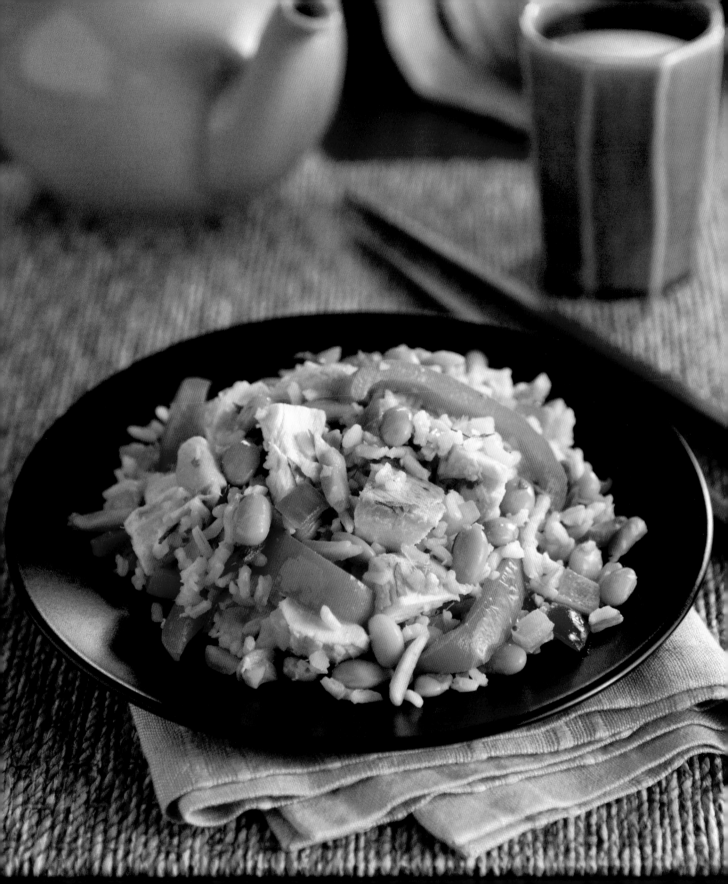

PASTA WITH TUNA, GREEN BEANS & TOMATOES

MAKES 6 SERVINGS

8 ounces uncooked whole wheat penne, rigatoni or fusilli pasta

1½ cups frozen cut green beans

3 teaspoons olive oil, divided

3 green onions, sliced

1 clove garlic, minced

1 can (about 14 ounces) diced Italian-style tomatoes, drained *or* 2 large tomatoes, chopped (about 2 cups)

½ teaspoon salt

½ teaspoon Italian seasoning

¼ teaspoon black pepper

1 can (12 ounces) solid albacore tuna packed in water, drained and flaked

Chopped fresh parsley (optional)

1. Cook pasta according to package directions, omitting salt and fat. Add green beans during last 7 minutes of cooking time (allow water to return to a boil before resuming timing). Drain and keep warm.

2. Meanwhile, heat 1 teaspoon oil in large skillet over medium heat. Add green onions and garlic; cook and stir 2 minutes. Add tomatoes, salt, Italian seasoning and pepper; cook and stir 4 to 5 minutes. Add pasta mixture, tuna and remaining 2 teaspoons oil; mix gently. Garnish with parsley. Serve immediately.

PER SERVING

CALORIES
228

TOTAL FAT
4g

SATURATED FAT
1g

CHOLESTEROL
14mg

SODIUM
345mg

CARBS
34g

DIETARY FIBER
3g

PROTEIN
15g

DIETARY EXCHANGES

2 bread/starch,
3 meat,
1 vegetable

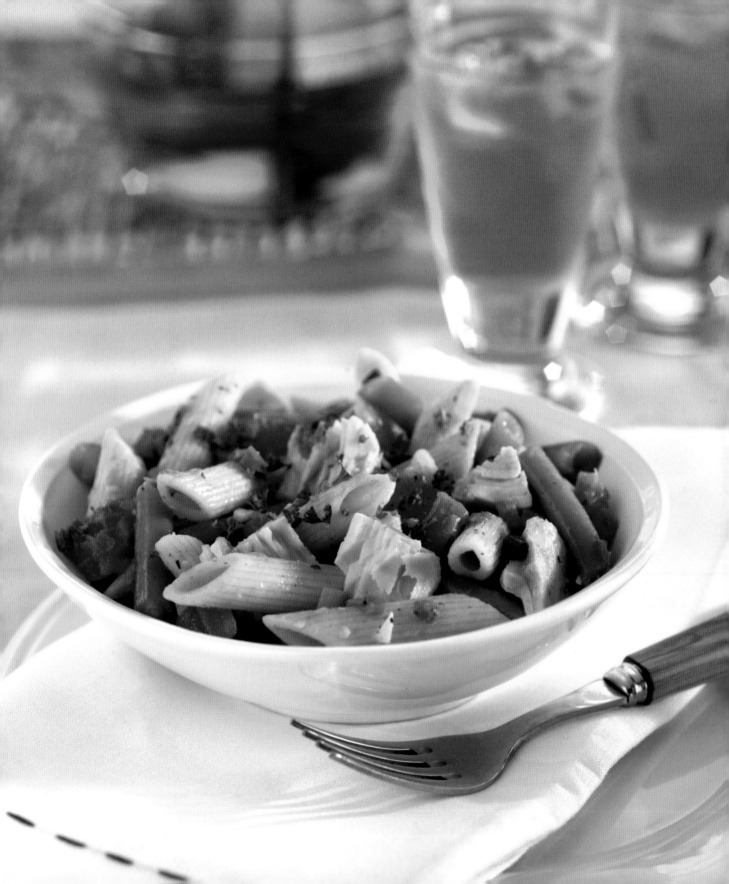

ORANGE TERIYAKI PORK

MAKES 4 SERVINGS

1 pound lean pork stew meat, cut into 1-inch cubes

1 package (16 ounces) frozen bell pepper blend for stir-fry

4 ounces sliced water chestnuts

½ cup orange juice

2 tablespoons quick-cooking tapioca

2 tablespoons packed light brown sugar

2 tablespoons teriyaki sauce

½ teaspoon ground ginger

½ teaspoon dry mustard

1⅓ cups hot cooked rice

Slow Cooker Directions

1. Spray large skillet with nonstick cooking spray; heat skillet over medium heat. Add pork; brown on all sides. Remove from heat; set aside.

2. Place bell peppers and water chestnuts in slow cooker. Top with browned pork. Mix orange juice, tapioca, brown sugar, teriyaki sauce, ginger and mustard in large bowl. Pour over pork mixture in slow cooker. Cover; cook on LOW 3 to 4 hours. Serve with rice.

PER SERVING

CALORIES
313

TOTAL FAT
6g

SATURATED FAT
2g

CHOLESTEROL
49mg

SODIUM
406mg

CARBS
42g

DIETARY FIBER
4g

PROTEIN
21g

DIETARY EXCHANGES

2 bread/starch,
2 meat,
2 vegetable

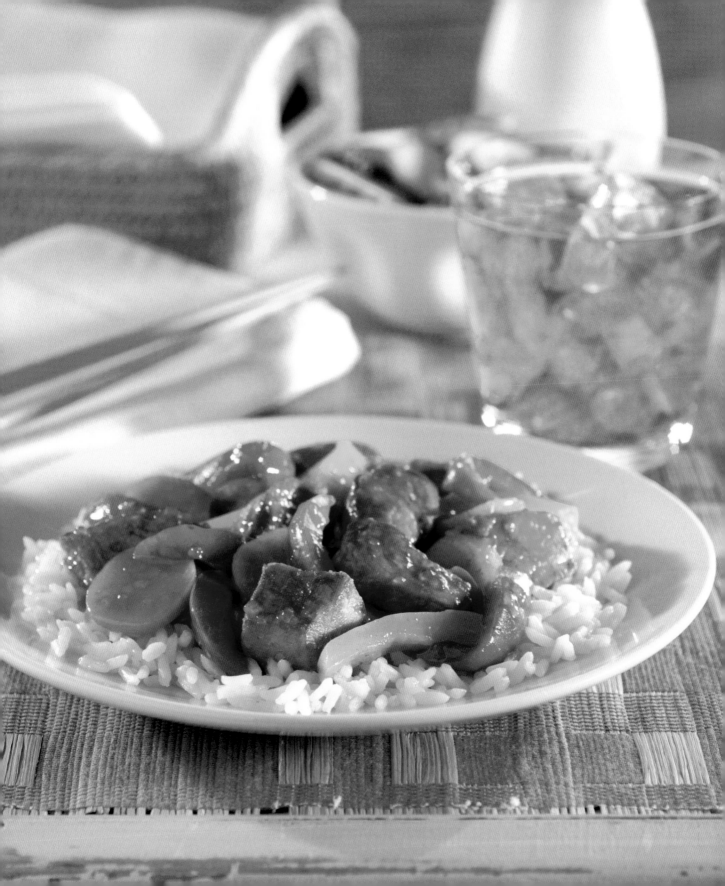

SHRIMP AND VEGGIE SKILLET TOSS

¼ cup reduced-sodium soy sauce

2 tablespoons lime juice

1 tablespoon sesame oil

1 teaspoon grated fresh ginger

⅛ teaspoon red pepper flakes

32 medium raw shrimp (about 8 ounces total), peeled, deveined, rinsed and patted dry (with tails on)

2 medium zucchini, cut in half lengthwise and thinly sliced

6 green onions, trimmed and halved lengthwise

12 grape tomatoes

1. Whisk soy sauce, lime juice, oil, ginger and red pepper flakes in small bowl; set aside.

2. Spray large nonstick skillet with nonstick cooking spray; heat over medium-high heat. Add shrimp; cook and stir 3 minutes or until shrimp are opaque. Remove from skillet.

3. Spray same skillet with cooking spray. Add zucchini; cook and stir 4 to 6 minutes or just until crisp-tender. Add green onions and tomatoes; cook 1 to 2 minutes. Add shrimp, cook 1 minute. Transfer to large bowl.

4. Add soy sauce mixture to skillet; bring to a boil. Remove from heat. Stir in shrimp and vegetables; gently toss.

Note

Shrimp are very low in calories and fat, and high in protein. They're also a good source of vitamin D and vitamin B12. All seafood are very sensitive to temperature, so return shrimp to refrigerator as soon as possible after purchasing.

PER SERVING

CALORIES
110

TOTAL FAT
4.5g

SATURATED FAT
0.5g

CHOLESTEROL
70mg

SODIUM
920mg

CARBS
10g

DIETARY FIBER
2g

PROTEIN
11g

DIETARY EXCHANGES

1 meat,
1½ vegetable,
½ fat

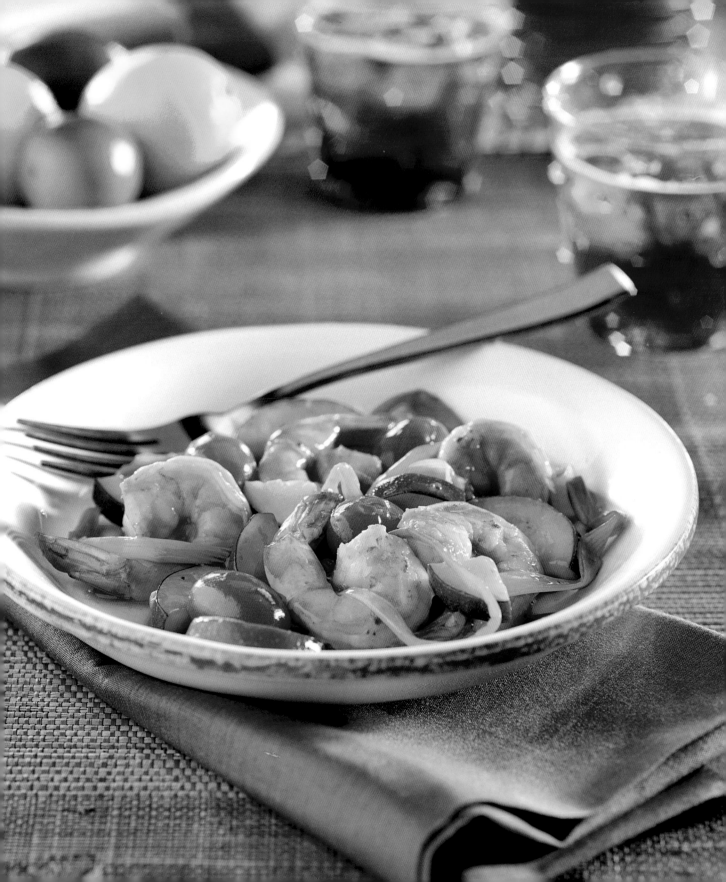

BAKED PASTA CASSEROLE

MAKES 2 SERVINGS

1½ cups (3 ounces) uncooked wagon wheel (rotelle) pasta

3 ounces 95% lean ground beef

2 tablespoons chopped onion

2 tablespoons chopped green bell pepper

1 clove garlic, minced

½ cup fat-free pasta sauce

Dash black pepper

2 tablespoons shredded Italian-style mozzarella and Parmesan cheese blend

1. Preheat oven to 350°F. Cook pasta according to package directions, omitting salt. Drain; return pasta to saucepan.

2. Meanwhile, heat medium nonstick skillet over medium-high heat. Add beef, onion, bell pepper and garlic; cook and stir 3 to 4 minutes or until beef is no longer pink and vegetables are crisp-tender. Drain.

3. Add beef mixture, pasta sauce and black pepper to pasta in saucepan; mix well. Spoon mixture into 1-quart baking dish. Sprinkle with cheese.

4. Bake 15 minutes or until heated through.

Note

To make ahead, assemble casserole as directed above through step 3. Cover and refrigerate several hours or overnight. Bake, uncovered, in preheated 350°F oven 30 minutes or until heated through.

PER SERVING

CALORIES
282

TOTAL FAT
7g

SATURATED FAT
3g

CHOLESTEROL
31mg

SODIUM
368mg

CARBS
37g

DIETARY FIBER
3g

PROTEIN
16g

DIETARY EXCHANGES

2 bread/starch,
1 meat,
2 vegetable,
1 fat

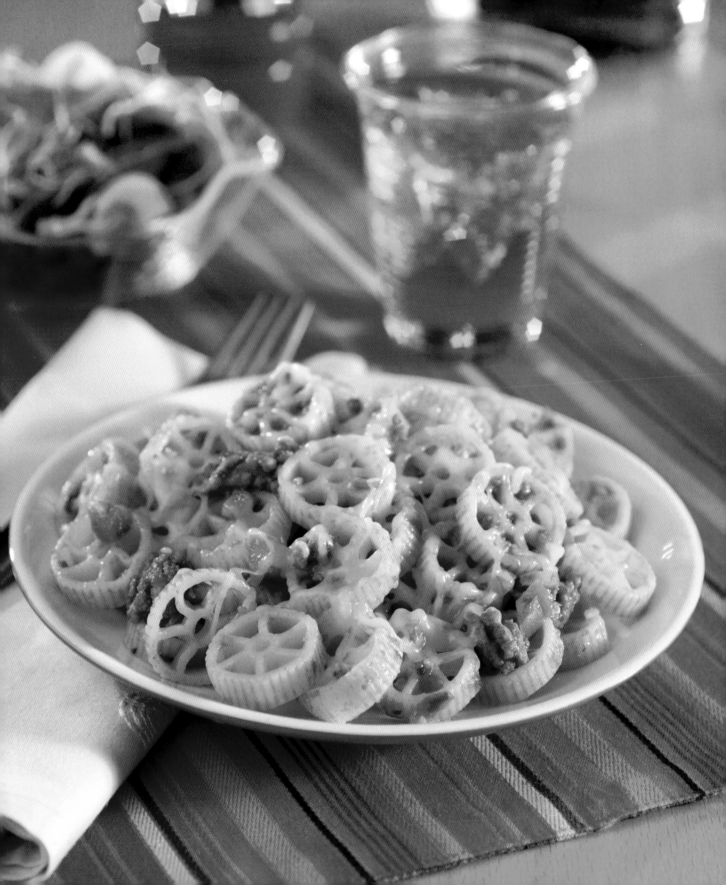

SAUERBRATEN

MAKES 5 SERVINGS

1 boneless beef rump roast (1¼ pounds)

3 cups baby carrots

1½ cups fresh or frozen pearl onions

¼ cup raisins

½ cup water

½ cup red wine vinegar

1 tablespoon honey

½ teaspoon salt

½ teaspoon dry mustard

½ teaspoon garlic-pepper seasoning

¼ teaspoon ground cloves

¼ cup crushed crisp gingersnap cookies (5 cookies)

Slow Cooker Directions

1. Heat large nonstick skillet over medium-high heat until hot. Brown roast on all sides. Place roast, carrots, onions and raisins in slow cooker.

2. Combine water, vinegar, honey, salt, mustard, garlic-pepper seasoning and cloves in large bowl; mix well. Pour mixture over meat and vegetables in slow cooker. Cover; cook on LOW 4 to 6 hours or until internal temperature reaches 145°F when tested with meat thermometer inserted into thickest part of roast.

3. Transfer roast to cutting board; cover with foil. Let stand 10 to 15 minutes before slicing. (Internal temperature will continue to rise 5° to 10°F during stand time.)

4. Remove vegetables from slow cooker with slotted spoon to bowl; cover to keep warm.

5. *Increase slow cooker temperature to HIGH.* Stir crushed cookies into sauce mixture in slow cooker. Cover; cook on HIGH 10 to 15 minutes or until sauce thickens. Serve meat and vegetables with sauce.

PER SERVING

CALORIES
296

TOTAL FAT
8g

SATURATED FAT
3g

CHOLESTEROL
57mg

SODIUM
381mg

CARBS
25g

DIETARY FIBER
4g

PROTEIN
28g

DIETARY EXCHANGES

½ bread/starch,
3 meat,
3 vegetable,
½ fruit

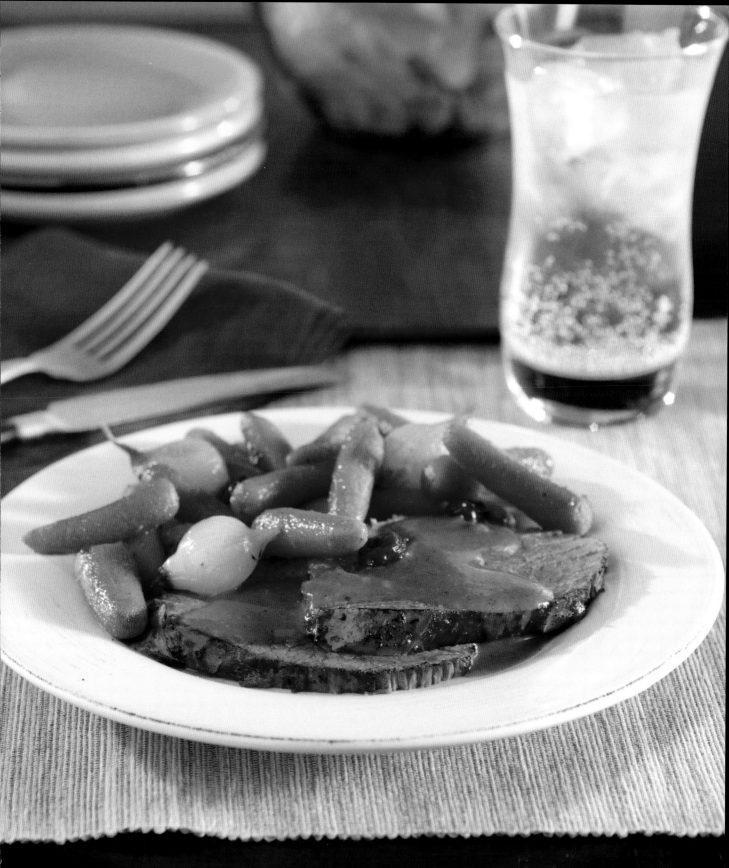

ROAST DILL SCROD WITH ASPARAGUS

MAKES 4 SERVINGS

1 bunch (12 ounces) asparagus spears, ends trimmed

1 teaspoon olive oil

4 scrod or cod fillets (about 5 ounces each)

1 tablespoon lemon juice

1 teaspoon dried dill weed

½ teaspoon salt

¼ teaspoon black pepper

Paprika (optional)

1. Preheat oven to 425°F.

2. Place asparagus in 13×9-inch baking dish; drizzle with oil. Roll asparagus to coat lightly with oil; push to edges of dish, stacking asparagus into two layers.

3. Arrange fish fillets in center of baking dish; drizzle with lemon juice. Combine dill weed, salt and pepper in small bowl; sprinkle over fish and asparagus. Sprinkle with paprika, if desired.

4. Roast 15 to 17 minutes or until asparagus is crisp-tender and fish is opaque in center and begins to flake when tested with fork.

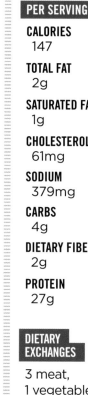

PER SERVING

CALORIES
147

TOTAL FAT
2g

SATURATED FAT
1g

CHOLESTEROL
61mg

SODIUM
379mg

CARBS
4g

DIETARY FIBER
2g

PROTEIN
27g

DIETARY EXCHANGES

3 meat,
1 vegetable

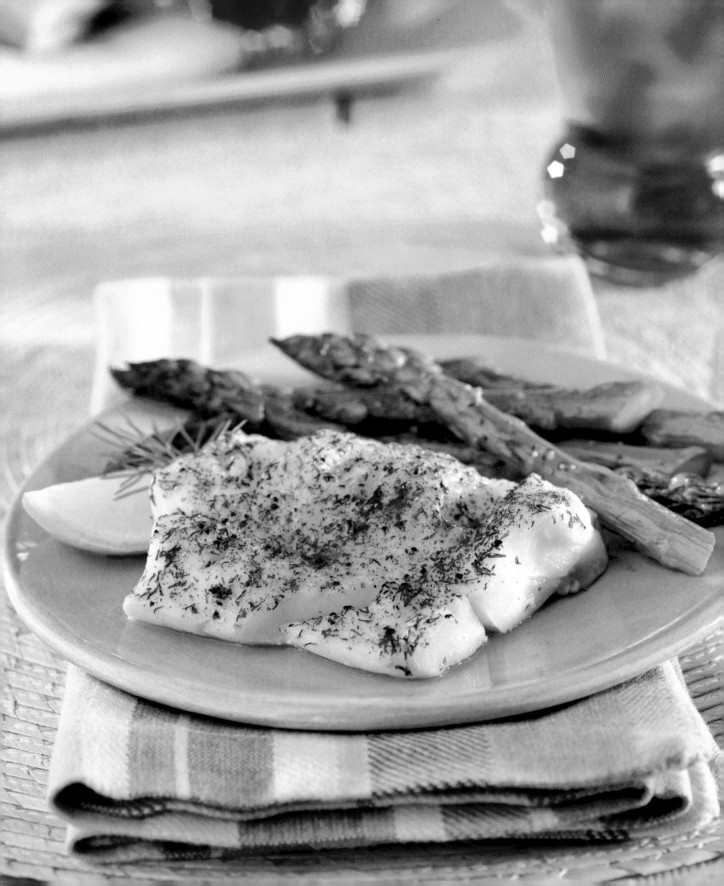

BOLOGNESE SAUCE & PENNE PASTA

MAKES 2 SERVINGS

½ **pound 95% lean ground beef**

⅓ **cup chopped onion**

1 **clove garlic, minced**

1 **can (8 ounces) tomato sauce**

⅓ **cup chopped carrot**

¼ **cup water**

2 **tablespoons dry red wine**

1 **teaspoon Italian seasoning**

1½ **cups hot cooked penne pasta**

Chopped fresh parsley

1. Brown beef, onion and garlic in medium saucepan over medium-high heat 6 to 8 minutes, stirring to break up meat. Drain fat.

2. Add tomato sauce, carrot, water, wine and Italian seasoning; bring to a boil. Reduce heat; simmer 15 minutes.

3. Serve sauce over pasta. Sprinkle with parsley.

PER SERVING

CALORIES
292

TOTAL FAT
5g

SATURATED FAT
2g

CHOLESTEROL
45mg

SODIUM
734mg

CARBS
40g

DIETARY FIBER
4g

PROTEIN
21g

DIETARY EXCHANGES

2 bread/starch,
2 meat,
1 vegetable

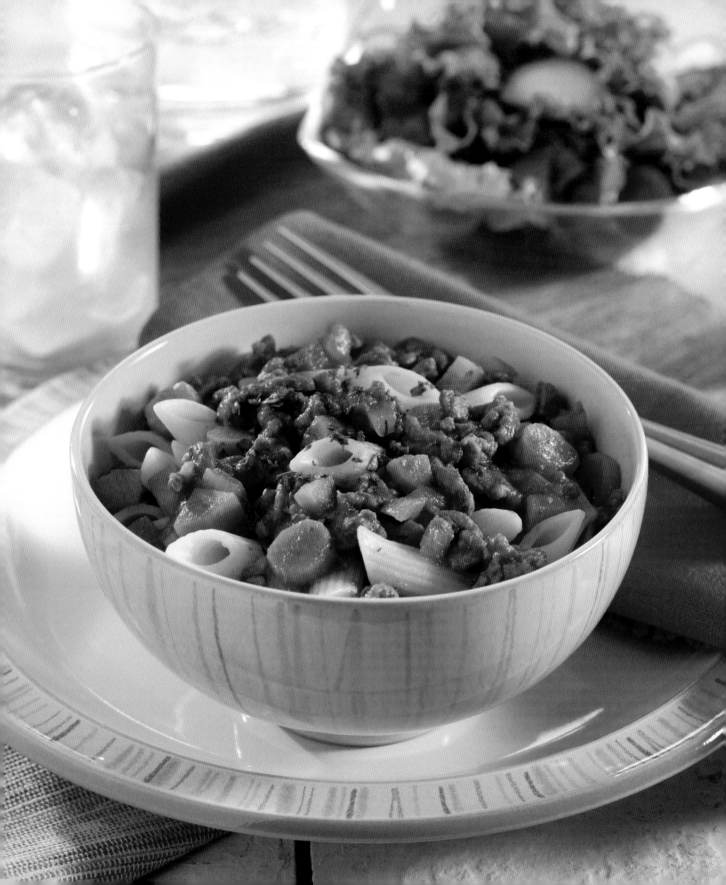

CHICKEN PICCATA

MAKES 4 SERVINGS

- 3 tablespoons all-purpose flour
- ½ teaspoon salt
- ¼ teaspoon black pepper
- 4 boneless skinless chicken breasts (4 ounces each)
- 2 teaspoons olive oil
- 1 teaspoon butter
- 2 cloves garlic, minced
- ¾ cup fat-free reduced-sodium chicken broth
- 1 tablespoon fresh lemon juice
- 2 tablespoons chopped fresh Italian parsley
- 1 tablespoon capers, drained

1. Combine flour, salt and pepper in shallow dish. Reserve 1 tablespoon flour mixture for sauce.

2. Pound chicken to ½-inch thickness between sheets of waxed paper with flat side of meat mallet or rolling pin. Coat chicken with remaining flour mixture, shaking off excess.

3. Heat oil and butter in large nonstick skillet over medium heat. Add chicken; cook 4 to 5 minutes per side or until no longer pink in center. Transfer to serving platter; cover loosely with foil.

4. Add garlic to skillet; cook and stir 1 minute. Add reserved flour mixture; cook and stir 1 minute. Add broth and lemon juice; cook 2 minutes or until sauce thickens, stirring frequently. Stir in parsley and capers; spoon sauce over chicken.

PER SERVING

CALORIES
194

TOTAL FAT
6g

SATURATED FAT
2g

CHOLESTEROL
71mg

SODIUM
473mg

CARBS
5g

DIETARY FIBER
1g

PROTEIN
27g

DIETARY EXCHANGES

½ bread/starch, 3 meat

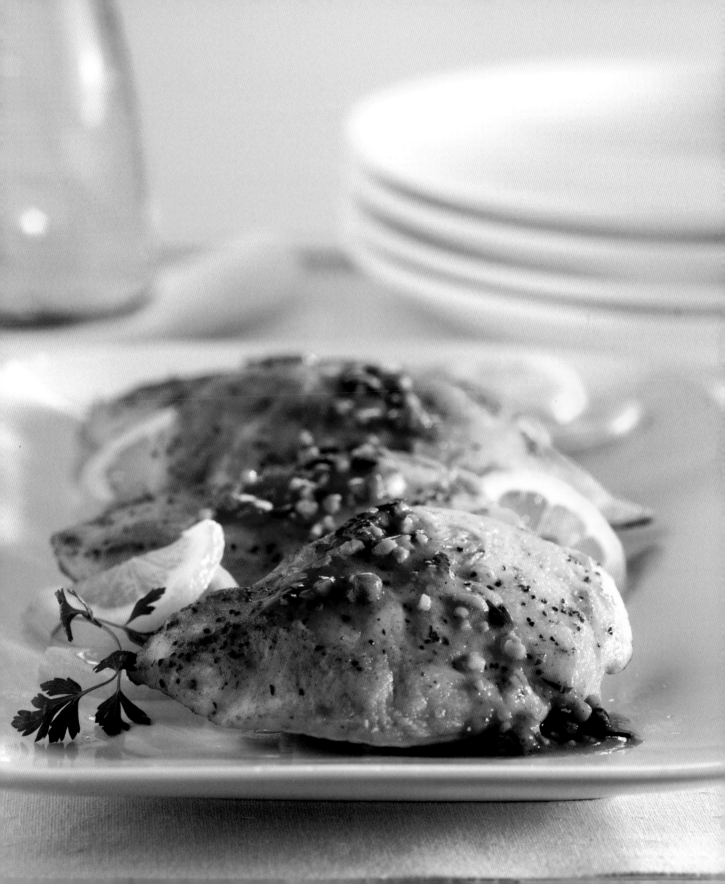

GREEK-STYLE BEEF KABOBS

MAKES 4 SERVINGS

- 1 **pound boneless beef top sirloin steak (1 inch thick), cut into 16 pieces**
- ¼ **cup fat-free Italian salad dressing**
- 3 **tablespoons fresh lemon juice, divided**
- 1 **tablespoon dried oregano**
- 1 **tablespoon Worcestershire sauce**
- 2 **teaspoons dried basil**
- 1 **teaspoon grated lemon peel**
- ⅛ **teaspoon red pepper flakes**
- 1 **large green bell pepper, cut into 16 pieces**
- 16 **cherry tomatoes**
- 2 **teaspoons olive oil**
- ⅛ **teaspoon salt**

1. Combine beef, salad dressing, 2 tablespoons lemon juice, oregano, Worcestershire sauce, basil, lemon peel and red pepper flakes in large resealable food storage bag. Seal bag; turn to coat. Marinate in refrigerator at least 8 hours or overnight, turning occasionally.

2. Preheat broiler. Remove beef from marinade; reserve marinade. Thread 4 (10-inch) skewers with beef, alternating with bell pepper and tomatoes. Spray rimmed baking sheet or broiler pan with nonstick cooking spray. Brush kabobs with marinade; place on baking sheet. Discard remaining marinade. Broil kabobs 3 minutes. Turn over; broil 2 minutes or until desired doneness is reached. ***Do not overcook.*** Remove skewers to serving platter.

3. Add remaining 1 tablespoon lemon juice, oil and salt to pan drippings on baking sheet; stir well, scraping bottom of pan with flat spatula. Pour juices over kabobs.

PER SERVING

CALORIES
193

TOTAL FAT
8g

SATURATED FAT
2g

CHOLESTEROL
69mg

SODIUM
159mg

CARBS
5g

DIETARY FIBER
1g

PROTEIN
25g

DIETARY EXCHANGES

3 meat,
1 vegetable

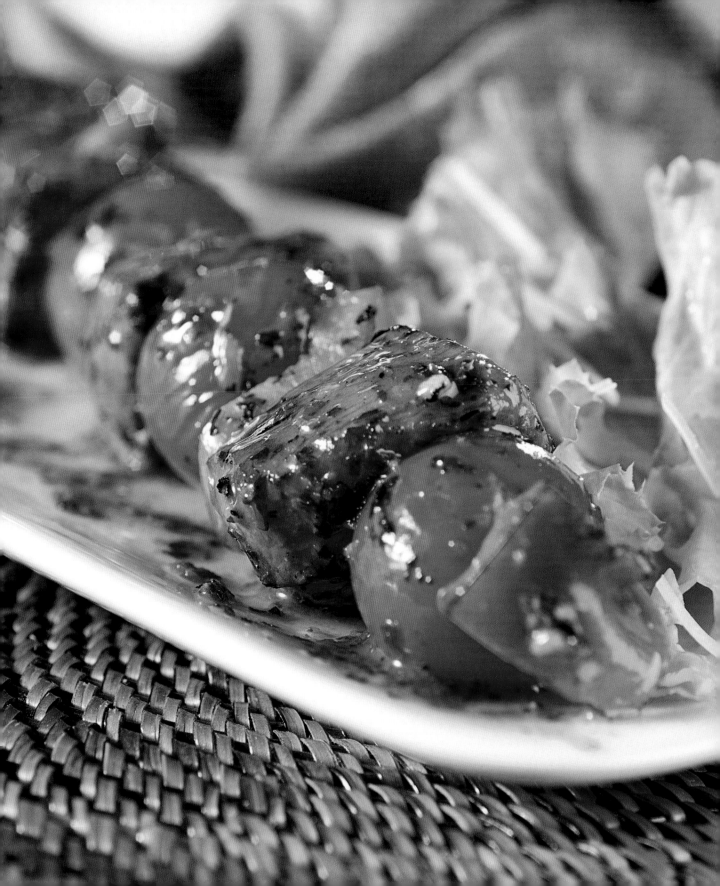

LEMON-GARLIC SALMON WITH TZATZIKI SAUCE

MAKES 4 SERVINGS

- ½ cup diced cucumber
- ¾ teaspoon salt, divided
- 1 cup plain nonfat Greek yogurt
- 2 tablespoons fresh lemon juice, divided
- 1 teaspoon grated lemon peel, divided
- 1 teaspoon minced garlic, divided
- ¼ teaspoon black pepper
- 4 skinless salmon fillets (4 ounces each)

1. Place cucumber in small colander set over small bowl; sprinkle with ¼ teaspoon salt. Drain 1 hour.

2. For tzatziki sauce, stir yogurt, cucumber, 1 tablespoon lemon juice, ½ teaspoon lemon peel, ½ teaspoon garlic and ¼ teaspoon salt in small bowl until combined. Cover and refrigerate until ready to use.

3. Combine remaining 1 tablespoon lemon juice, ½ teaspoon lemon peel, ½ teaspoon garlic, ¼ teaspoon salt and pepper in small bowl; mix well. Rub evenly onto salmon.

4. Heat nonstick grill pan over medium-high heat. Cook salmon 5 minutes per side or until fish begins to flake when tested with fork. Serve with tzatziki sauce.

Serving Suggestion

Serve this Mediterranean-inspired dish with fresh vegetables or a savory salad, if desired.

PER SERVING

CALORIES
243

TOTAL FAT
12g

SATURATED FAT
2g

CHOLESTEROL
60mg

SODIUM
508mg

CARBS
3g

DIETARY FIBER
0g

PROTEIN
29g

DIETARY EXCHANGES

3 meat,
1 vegetable

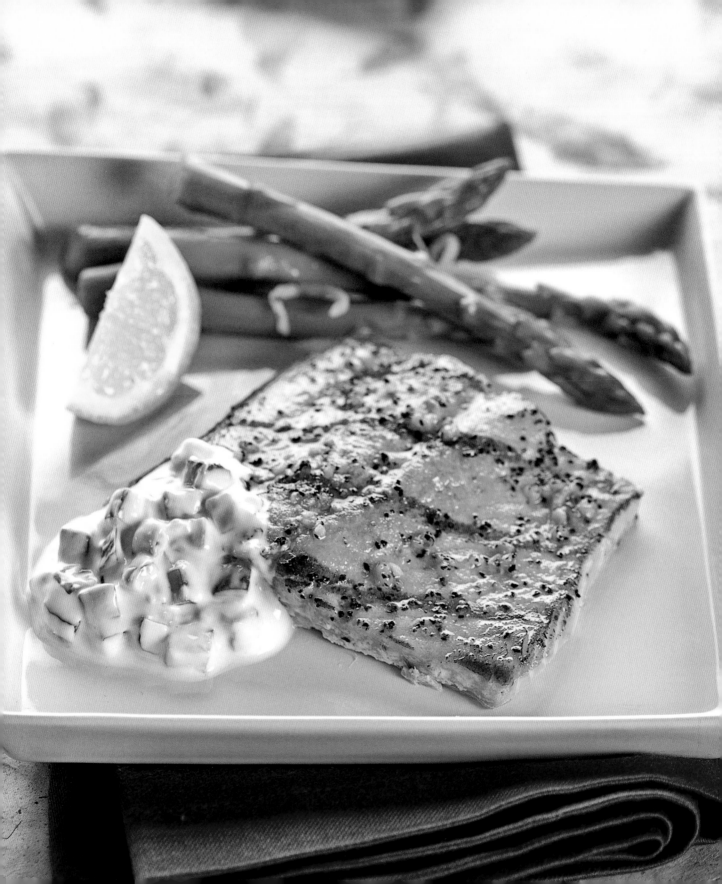

TURKEY SAUSAGE & SPINACH STUFFED SHELLS

MAKES 6 SERVINGS (3 FILLED SHELLS EACH)

- 18 uncooked jumbo shell pasta
- 1 teaspoon olive oil
- 8 ounces spicy Italian turkey sausage, casings removed
- ½ cup chopped onion
- 2 cloves garlic, minced
- 1 package (6 ounces) baby spinach
- 1 cup fat-free ricotta cheese
- 1½ cups tomato-basil pasta sauce, divided
- ½ cup shredded Parmesan cheese, divided
- ¼ cup chopped fresh basil

1. Preheat oven to 375°F. Cook pasta according to package directions; drain.

2. Meanwhile, heat oil in large nonstick skillet over medium heat. Add sausage, onion and garlic; cook 5 minutes or until sausage begins to brown, stirring to break up meat. Add spinach in batches; cook and stir until wilted. Remove from heat; stir in ricotta cheese, ½ cup pasta sauce and ¼ cup Parmesan cheese.

3. Arrange shells in 2-quart casserole. Fill shells evenly with turkey mixture. Spoon remaining 1 cup pasta sauce evenly over shells. Cover with foil.

4. Bake 30 to 35 minutes or until heated through. Top with remaining ¼ cup Parmesan cheese and basil.

PER SERVING

CALORIES
255

TOTAL FAT
5g

SATURATED FAT
2g

CHOLESTEROL
24mg

SODIUM
580mg

CARBS
36g

DIETARY FIBER
4g

PROTEIN
15g

DIETARY EXCHANGES

2 bread/starch,
1 meat,
1 vegetable,
½ fat

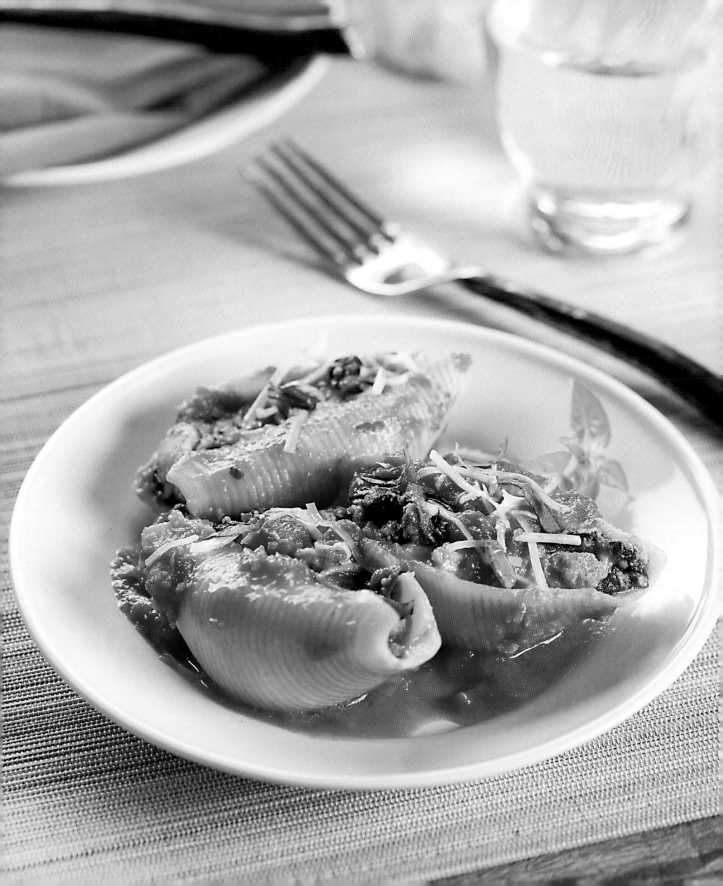

MINI MEATLOAVES

MAKES 6 SERVINGS

- 3 tablespoons ketchup
- 1 tablespoon balsamic vinegar
- 1 tablespoon olive oil
- 1½ cups finely chopped onion
- 1½ cups finely chopped mushrooms
- 1½ cups chopped baby spinach
- 1½ pounds extra lean ground sirloin
- ¾ cup old-fashioned oats
- 2 egg whites
- ½ teaspoon salt
- ½ teaspoon black pepper

1. Preheat oven to 375°F. Spray 6 mini (4¼×2½-inch) loaf pans with nonstick cooking spray. Whisk ketchup and vinegar in small bowl until smooth and well blended; set aside.

2. Heat oil in large skillet over medium heat. Add onion, mushrooms and spinach; cook and stir 8 minutes or until tender. Remove to large bowl. Let stand until cool enough to handle.

3. Add beef, oats, egg whites, salt and pepper to vegetables; mix well. Divide mixture evenly among prepared pans. Brush half of ketchup mixture evenly over loaves.

4. Bake 15 minutes. Brush with remaining ketchup mixture. Bake 5 minutes or until cooked through (160°F).

PER SERVING

CALORIES
270

TOTAL FAT
11g

SATURATED FAT
3g

CHOLESTEROL
62mg

SODIUM
362mg

CARBS
14g

DIETARY FIBER
2g

PROTEIN
28g

DIETARY EXCHANGES

1 bread/starch, 3½ meat

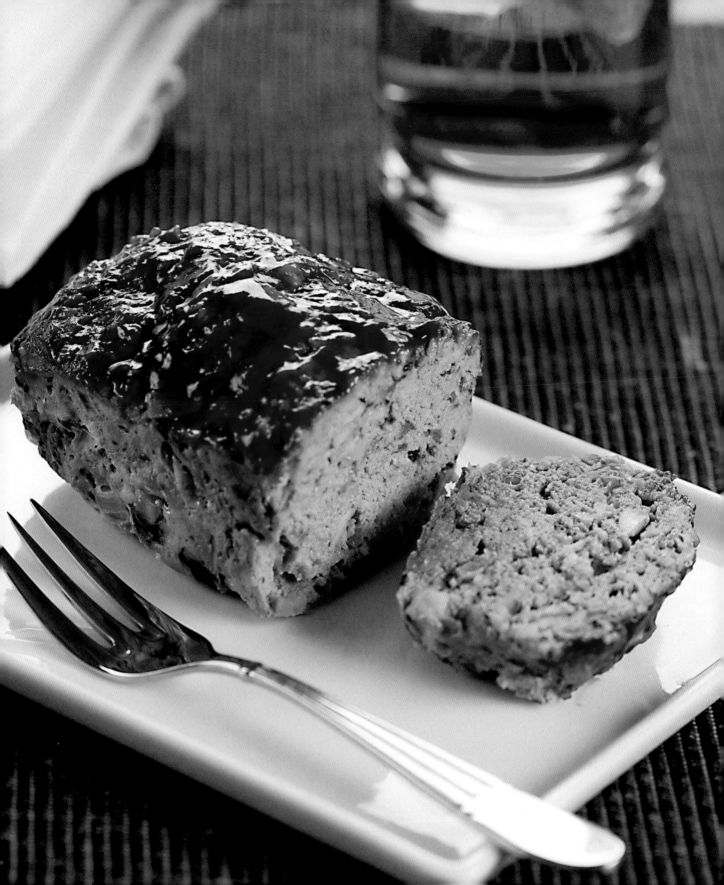

EASY SEAFOOD STIR-FRY

MAKES 4 SERVINGS

- 1 package (1 ounce) dried black Chinese mushrooms*
- ½ cup fat-free reduced-sodium chicken broth
- 2 tablespoons dry sherry
- 1 tablespoon reduced-sodium soy sauce
- 4½ teaspoons cornstarch
- 1 teaspoon vegetable oil, divided
- 8 ounces bay scallops or halved sea scallops
- 4 ounces medium raw shrimp, peeled and deveined
- 2 cloves garlic, minced
- 6 ounces (2 cups) fresh snow peas, cut diagonally into halves
- 2 cups hot cooked rice
- ¼ cup thinly sliced green onions

Or substitute 1½ cups sliced mushrooms and omit step 1.

1. Place mushrooms in medium bowl; cover with warm water. Soak 20 to 40 minutes or until soft. Drain and squeeze out excess water. Discard stems; thinly slice caps.

2. Whisk broth, sherry, soy sauce and cornstarch in small bowl until smooth.

3. Heat ½ teaspoon oil in wok or large nonstick skillet over medium heat. Add scallops, shrimp and garlic; stir-fry 3 minutes or until seafood is opaque. Remove to large plate.

4. Heat remaining ½ teaspoon oil in wok. Add mushrooms and snow peas; stir-fry 3 minutes or until snow peas are crisp-tender. Stir broth mixture; add to wok. Stir-fry 2 minutes or until sauce boils and thickens.

5. Return seafood and any accumulated juices to wok; stir-fry until heated through. Serve with rice; sprinkle with green onions.

PER SERVING

CALORIES
304

TOTAL FAT
3g

SATURATED FAT
1g

CHOLESTEROL
74mg

SODIUM
335mg

CARBS
42g

DIETARY FIBER
3g

PROTEIN
25g

DIETARY EXCHANGES

2 bread/starch, 2 meat, 2 vegetable

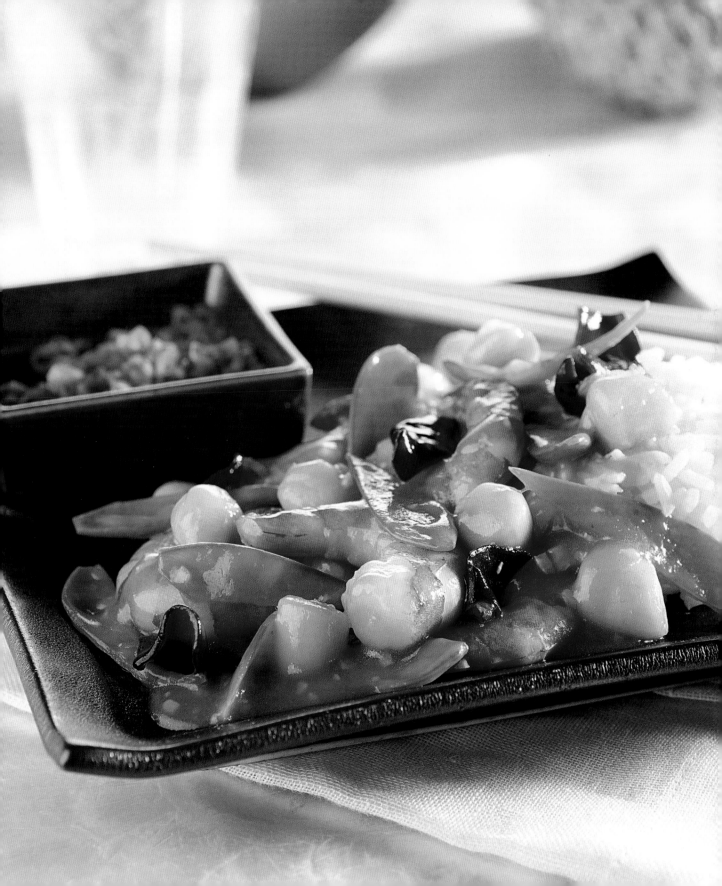

KALE & MUSHROOM STUFFED CHICKEN BREASTS

MAKES 4 SERVINGS

3 teaspoons olive oil, divided

1 cup coarsely chopped mushrooms

2 cups thinly sliced kale

1 tablespoon fresh lemon juice

½ teaspoon salt, divided

4 boneless skinless chicken breasts (about 4 ounces each)

¼ cup (1 ounce) crumbled fat-free feta cheese

¼ teaspoon black pepper

1. Heat 1 teaspoon oil in large skillet over medium-high heat. Add mushrooms; cook and stir 5 minutes or until mushrooms begin to brown. Add kale; cook and stir 8 minutes or until wilted. Sprinkle with lemon juice and ¼ teaspoon salt. Remove to small bowl. Let stand 5 to 10 minutes to cool slightly.

2. Meanwhile, place each chicken breast between sheets of plastic wrap. Pound with meat mallet or rolling pin to about ½-inch thickness.

3. Gently stir feta cheese into mushroom and kale mixture. Spoon ¼ cup mixture down center of each chicken breast. Roll up to enclose filling; secure with toothpicks. Sprinkle with remaining ¼ teaspoon salt and pepper.

4. Wipe out same skillet with paper towels. Add remaining 2 teaspoons oil to skillet; heat over medium heat. Add chicken; brown on all sides. Cover and cook 5 minutes per side or until no longer pink. Remove toothpicks before serving.

PER SERVING

CALORIES
192

TOTAL FAT
7g

SATURATED FAT
1g

CHOLESTEROL
73mg

SODIUM
495mg

CARBS
4g

DIETARY FIBER
1g

PROTEIN
29g

DIETARY EXCHANGES

3 meat,
1 vegetable

Serving Suggestion

Serve this flavorful entrée with a fresh salad or summer vegetables.

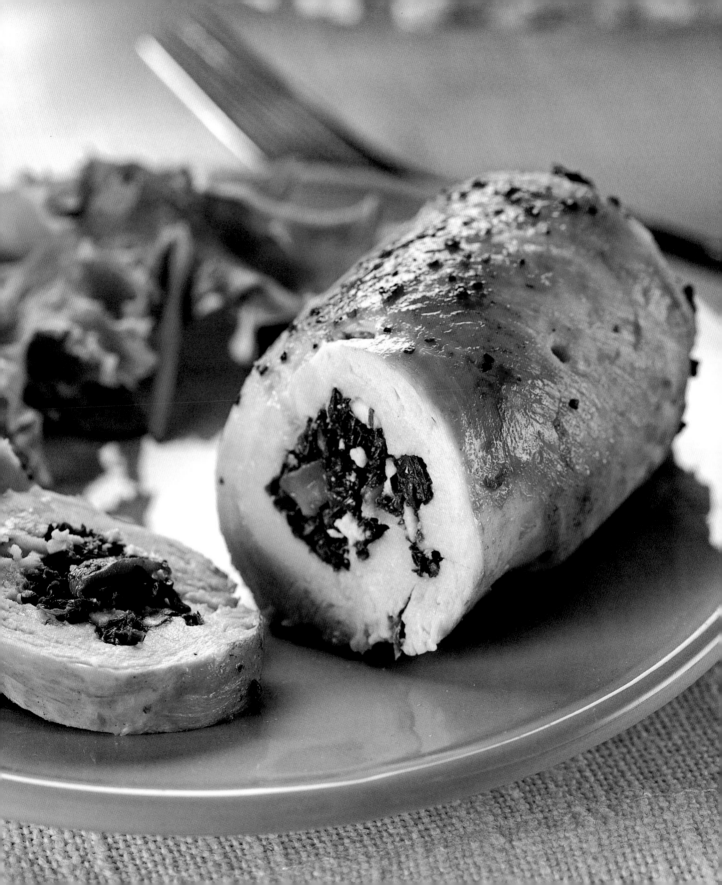

APRICOT BRISKET

MAKES 8 SERVINGS

1 cup chopped dried apricots, divided

1 cup canned diced tomatoes, divided

2 teaspoons ground cumin

1 teaspoon salt, divided

1 clove garlic

¼ teaspoon ground cinnamon

1 medium onion, thinly sliced

2 large carrots, cut into 1-inch pieces

1 small beef brisket (about 2 to 3 pounds), trimmed of fat

½ teaspoon black pepper

1½ cups low-sodium beef broth

2 tablespoons cold water

2 tablespoons cornstarch

Chopped fresh parsley (optional)

1. Preheat oven to 325°F.

2. Combine ½ cup chopped apricots, ½ cup tomatoes, cumin, ½ teaspoon salt, garlic and cinnamon in food processor. Process using on/off pulses until coarsely combined.

3. Place onion and carrots on bottom of roasting pan. Place brisket on top. Cut several small slits across top of brisket; gently spoon apricot mixture into slits. Sprinkle brisket with remaining ½ teaspoon salt and pepper. Spread remaining ½ cup diced tomatoes over brisket; top with remaining ½ cup apricots. Drizzle broth over brisket. Cover with foil.

4. Roast 2 to 2½ hours. Transfer brisket to carving board; tent with foil and let stand 15 minutes.

5. Pour pan juices and vegetables into medium saucepan. Stir water into cornstarch in small bowl until smooth and well blended. Stir into pan juices; simmer about 5 minutes or until thickened.

6. Carve brisket crosswise into thin slices; serve with onion, carrots, tomatoes, apricots and pan juices. Sprinkle with parsley, if desired.

PER SERVING

CALORIES
177

TOTAL FAT
4g

SATURATED FAT
1g

CHOLESTEROL
53mg

SODIUM
380mg

CARBS
17g

DIETARY FIBER
2g

PROTEIN
20g

DIETARY EXCHANGES

3 meat

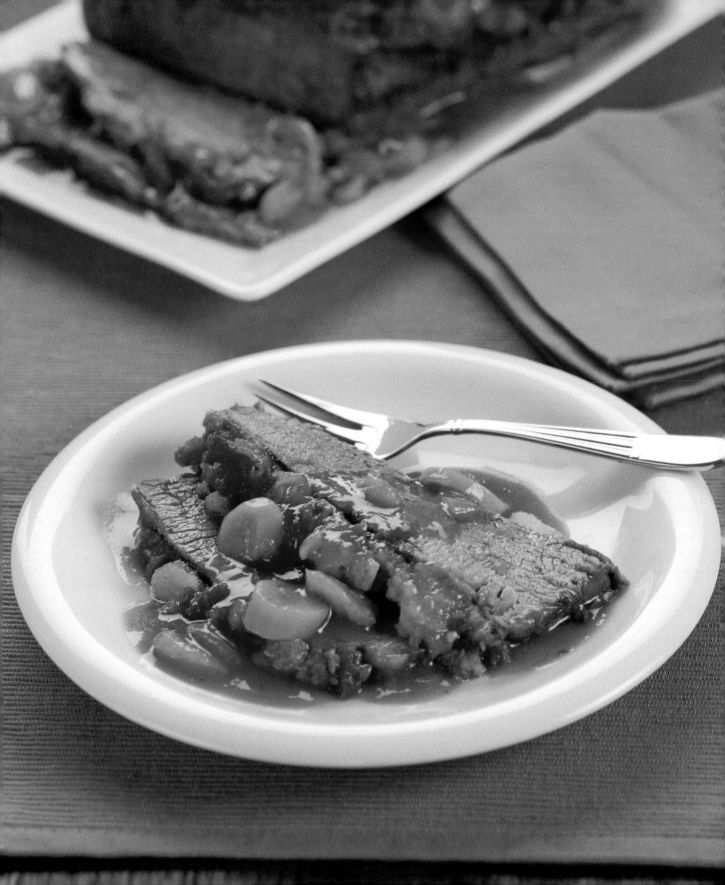

PORK AND PLUM KABOBS

MAKES 4 SERVINGS

- ¾ **pound boneless pork loin chops (1 inch thick), trimmed and cut into 1-inch pieces**
- 1½ **teaspoons ground cumin**
- ½ **teaspoon ground cinnamon**
- ¼ **teaspoon salt**
- ¼ **teaspoon garlic powder**
- ¼ **teaspoon ground red pepper**
- ¼ **cup sliced green onions**
- ¼ **cup raspberry fruit spread**
- 1 **tablespoon orange juice**
- 3 **plums or nectarines, pitted and cut into wedges**

1. Place pork in large resealable food storage bag. Combine cumin, cinnamon, salt, garlic powder and ground red pepper in small bowl; pour over pork. Seal bag; shake to coat meat with spices.

2. Combine green onions, fruit spread and orange juice in small bowl; set aside.

3. Prepare grill for direct cooking. Alternately thread pork and plum wedges onto 8 skewers.* Grill kabobs over medium heat 12 to 14 minutes or until meat is cooked through, turning once. Brush frequently with raspberry mixture during last 5 minutes of grilling.

If using wood skewers, soak in warm water 30 minutes to prevent burning.

Serving Suggestion

A crisp, cool salad makes a great accompaniment to these sweet grilled kabobs.

PER SERVING

CALORIES
191

TOTAL FAT
5g

SATURATED FAT
2g

CHOLESTEROL
53mg

SODIUM
183mg

CARBS
17g

DIETARY FIBER
1g

PROTEIN
19g

DIETARY EXCHANGES

3 meat,
1 fruit

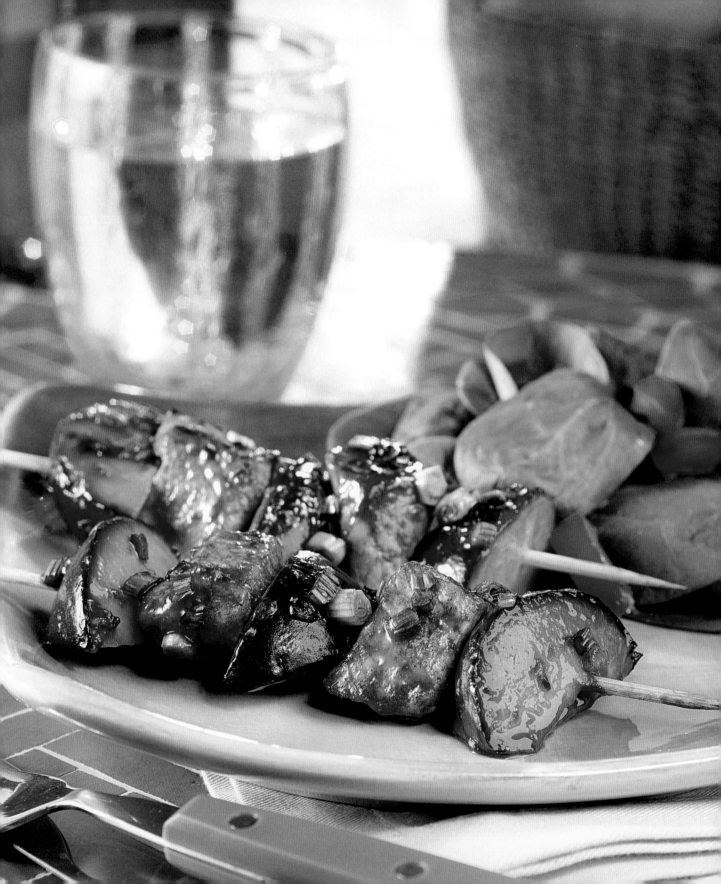

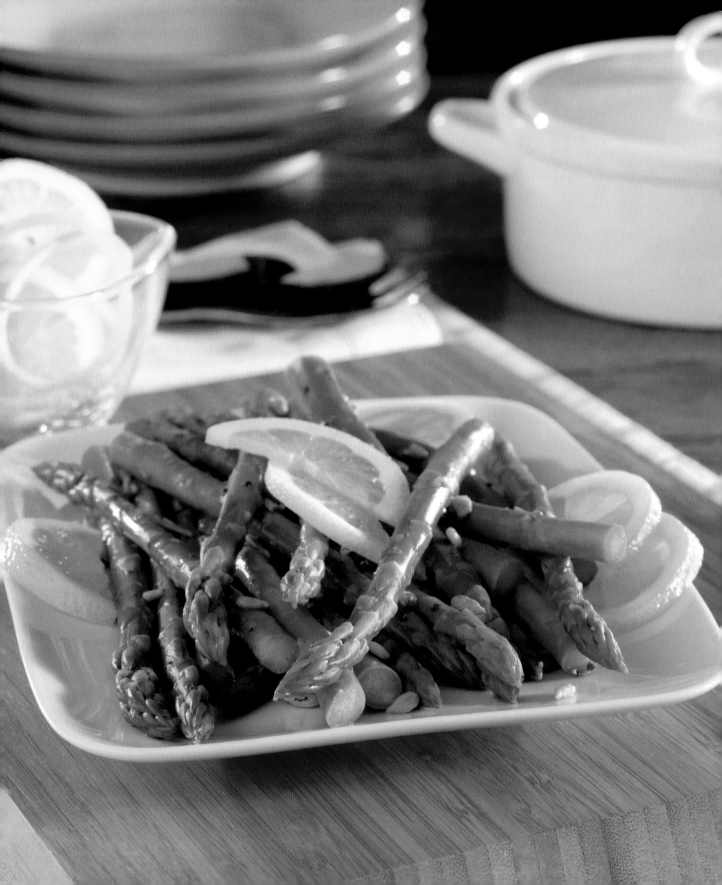

PICK A SIDE

CRUNCHY ASPARAGUS

MAKES 4 SERVINGS

1 package (10 ounces) frozen asparagus cuts

1 teaspoon lemon juice

3 to 4 drops hot pepper sauce

¼ teaspoon salt (optional)

¼ teaspoon dried basil

⅛ teaspoon black pepper

2 teaspoons sunflower kernels

Lemon slices (optional)

Microwave Directions

1. Place asparagus and 2 tablespoons water in 1-quart microwavable casserole dish; cover. Microwave on HIGH 4½ to 5½ minutes or until asparagus is hot, stirring halfway through cooking time to break apart. Drain. Cover; set aside.

2. Combine lemon juice, hot pepper sauce, salt, if desired, basil and pepper in small bowl. Pour mixture over asparagus; toss to coat. Sprinkle with sunflower kernels. Garnish with lemon slices, if desired.

PER SERVING

CALORIES
29

TOTAL FAT
1g

SATURATED FAT
1g

CHOLESTEROL
0mg

SODIUM
4mg

CARBS
4g

DIETARY FIBER
1g

PROTEIN
2g

DIETARY EXCHANGES

1 vegetable

CREAMY COLESLAW

½ **cup light mayonnaise**

½ **cup low-fat buttermilk**

2 **teaspoons sugar**

1 **teaspoon celery seed**

1 **teaspoon fresh lime juice**

½ **teaspoon chili powder**

3 **cups shredded coleslaw mix**

1 **cup shredded carrots**

¼ **cup finely chopped red onion**

Whisk mayonnaise, buttermilk, sugar, celery seed, lime juice and chili powder in large bowl until smooth and well blended. Add coleslaw mix, carrots and onion; toss to coat evenly. Cover and refrigerate at least 2 hours before serving.

PER SERVING

CALORIES
59

TOTAL FAT
4g

SATURATED FAT
1g

CHOLESTEROL
3mg

SODIUM
143mg

CARBS
6g

DIETARY FIBER
1g

PROTEIN
1g

DIETARY EXCHANGES

1 vegetable, 1 fat

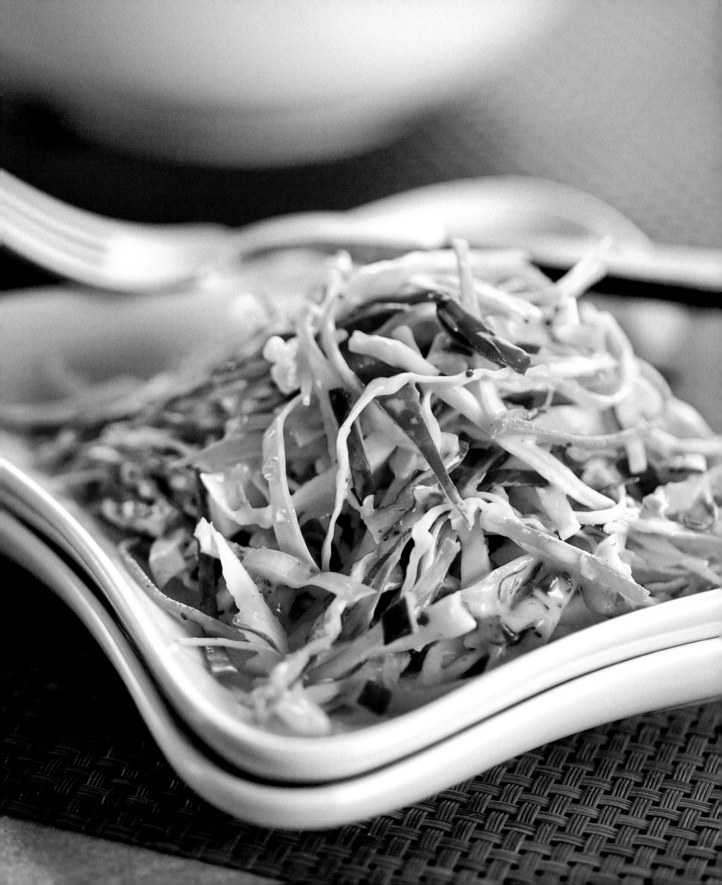

ROASTED BEET RISOTTO

MAKES 4 SERVINGS

2 medium beets, trimmed

4 cups vegetable broth

1 tablespoon canola oil

1 cup uncooked arborio rice

1 leek, finely chopped

½ cup crumbled goat cheese, plus additional for garnish

1 teaspoon Italian seasoning

¼ teaspoon salt

Juice of 1 lemon

Lemon wedges (optional)

1. Preheat oven to 400°F. Wrap each beet tightly in foil. Place on baking sheet. Roast 45 minutes to 1 hour or until knife inserted into centers goes in easily. Unwrap beets; discard foil. Let stand 15 minutes or until cool enough to handle. Peel and cut beets into bite-size pieces. Set aside.

2. Heat broth to a simmer in medium saucepan; keep warm.

3. Heat oil in large saucepan over medium-high heat. Add rice; cook and stir 1 to 2 minutes. Add leek; cook and stir 1 to 2 minutes. Add broth, ½ cup at a time, stirring constantly until broth is absorbed before adding next ½ cup. Continue adding broth and stirring until rice is tender and mixture is creamy, about 20 to 25 minutes. Remove from heat.

4. Stir ½ cup goat cheese, Italian seasoning and salt into risotto. Gently stir in beets. Sprinkle with lemon juice and additional cheese, if desired. Garnish with lemon wedges. Serve immediately.

PER SERVING

CALORIES
278

TOTAL FAT
8g

SATURATED FAT
3g

CHOLESTEROL
9mg

SODIUM
383mg

CARBS
45g

DIETARY FIBER
2g

PROTEIN
8g

DIETARY EXCHANGES

3 bread/starch, 2 fat

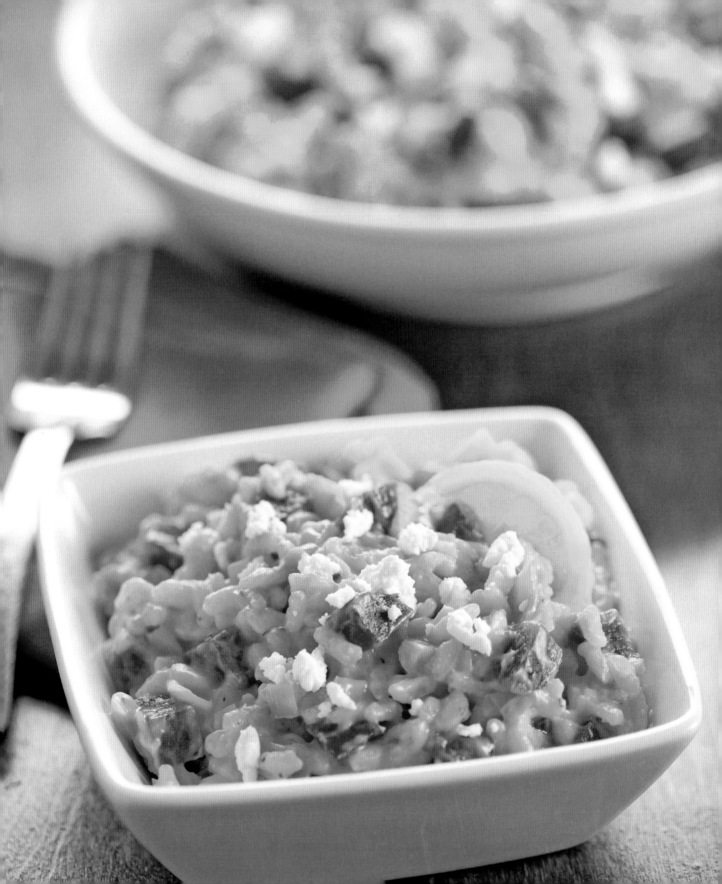

CARAMELIZED BRUSSELS SPROUTS WITH CRANBERRIES

MAKES 4 SERVINGS

1 tablespoon vegetable oil

1 pound Brussels sprouts, ends trimmed, thinly sliced

¼ cup dried cranberries

2 teaspoons packed brown sugar

¼ teaspoon salt

1. Heat oil in large skillet over medium-high heat. Add Brussels sprouts; cook 10 minutes or until crisp-tender and beginning to brown, stirring occasionally.

2. Add cranberries, brown sugar and salt; cook and stir 5 minutes or until Brussels sprouts are browned.

PER SERVING

CALORIES
105

TOTAL FAT
4g

SATURATED FAT
1g

CHOLESTEROL
0mg

SODIUM
317mg

CARBS
17g

DIETARY FIBER
4g

PROTEIN
3g

DIETARY EXCHANGES

2 vegetable, ½ fruit, ½ fat

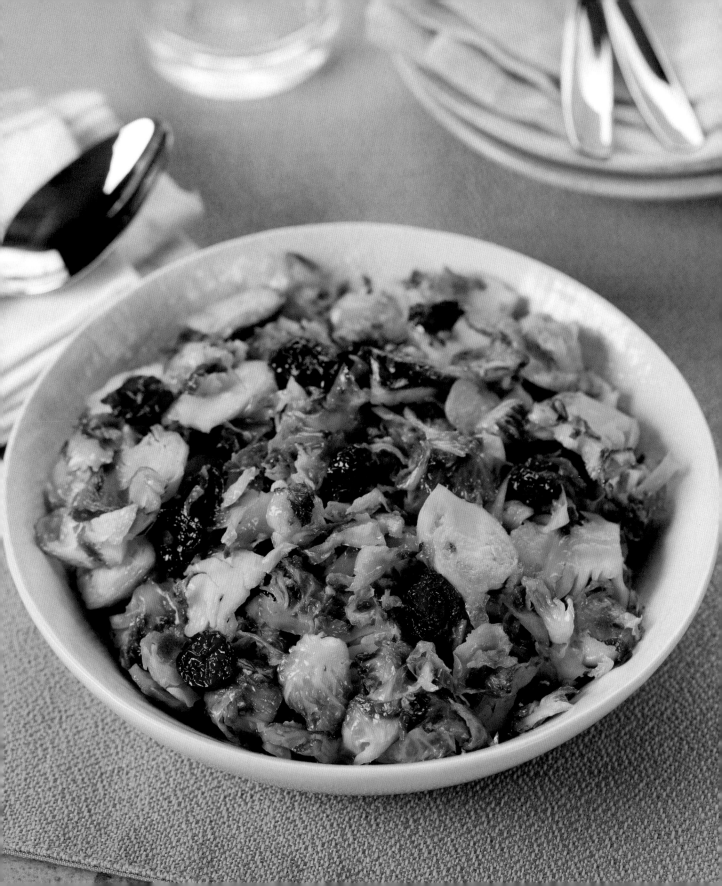

CAULIFLOWER POTATO PANCAKES

MAKES 12 PANCAKES (ABOUT 6 SERVINGS)

1½ cups cubed Yukon Gold potatoes, peeled

3 cups roughly chopped cauliflower

⅓ cup whole wheat flour

1 egg, lightly beaten

1 egg white

1 tablespoon chopped fresh chives, plus additional for garnish

1 teaspoon baking powder

½ teaspoon salt

3 teaspoons vegetable oil, divided

Light sour cream (optional)

1. Bring large saucepan of water to a boil. Add potatoes and cauliflower; reduce heat. Simmer 10 minutes or until fork-tender. Drain potatoes and cauliflower. Let stand 5 to 10 minutes or until cool enough to handle.

2. Gently mash potatoes and cauliflower in large bowl. Add flour, egg, egg white, 1 tablespoon chives, baking powder and salt; mix well.

3. Heat 1 teaspoon oil in large nonstick skillet over medium heat. Drop ¼ cupfuls potato mixture into skillet; flatten slightly. Cook 5 to 7 minutes per side or until golden brown. Repeat with remaining oil and potato mixture.

4. Serve with sour cream, if desired. Garnish with additional chives.

PER SERVING

CALORIES
89

TOTAL FAT
4g

SATURATED FAT
1g

CHOLESTEROL
31mg

SODIUM
313mg

CARBS
14g

DIETARY FIBER
2g

PROTEIN
4g

DIETARY EXCHANGES

½ bread/starch, 1 vegetable, ½ fat

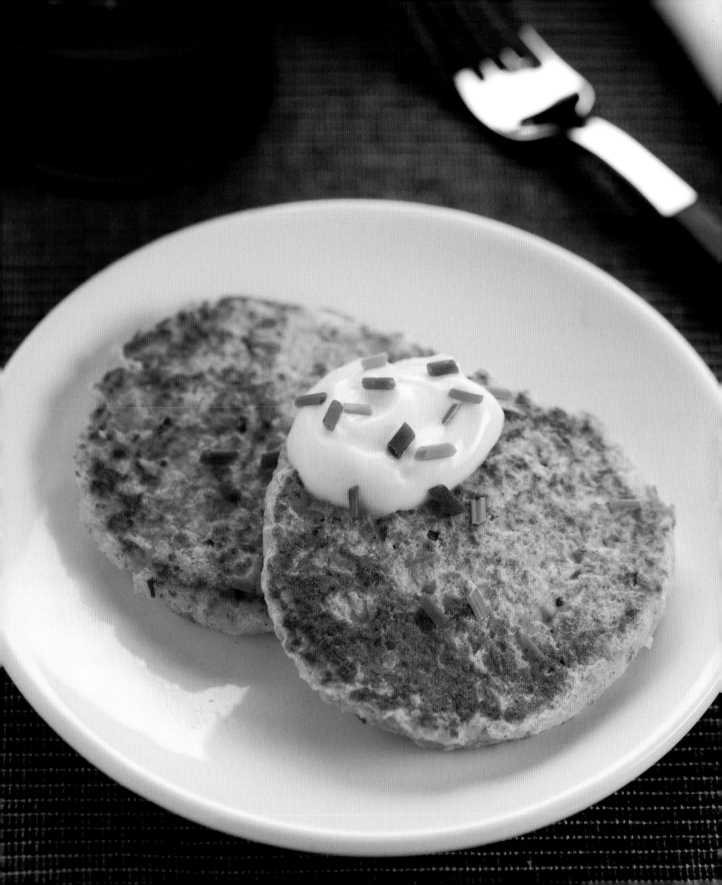

FRUIT & NUT QUINOA

MAKES 6 SERVINGS

1 cup uncooked quinoa

2 cups water

2 tablespoons finely grated orange peel, plus additional for garnish

¼ cup fresh orange juice

2 teaspoons olive oil

½ teaspoon salt

¼ teaspoon ground cinnamon

⅓ cup dried cranberries

⅓ cup toasted pistachio nuts*

To toast pistachios, spread in single layer in heavy skillet. Cook and stir over medium heat 1 to 2 minutes or until nuts are lightly browned.

1. Place quinoa in fine-mesh strainer; rinse well under cold running water.

2. Bring 2 cups water to a boil in medium saucepan over high heat; stir in quinoa. Reduce heat to low; cover and simmer 10 to 15 minutes or until quinoa is tender and water is absorbed. Stir in 2 tablespoons orange peel.

3. Whisk orange juice, oil, salt and cinnamon in small bowl. Pour over quinoa; gently toss to coat. Fold in cranberries and pistachios. Serve warm or at room temperature. Garnish with additional orange peel.

PER SERVING

CALORIES
185

TOTAL FAT
6g

SATURATED FAT
1g

CHOLESTEROL
0mg

SODIUM
198mg

CARBS
27g

DIETARY FIBER
3g

PROTEIN
5g

DIETARY EXCHANGES

2 bread/starch, 1 fat

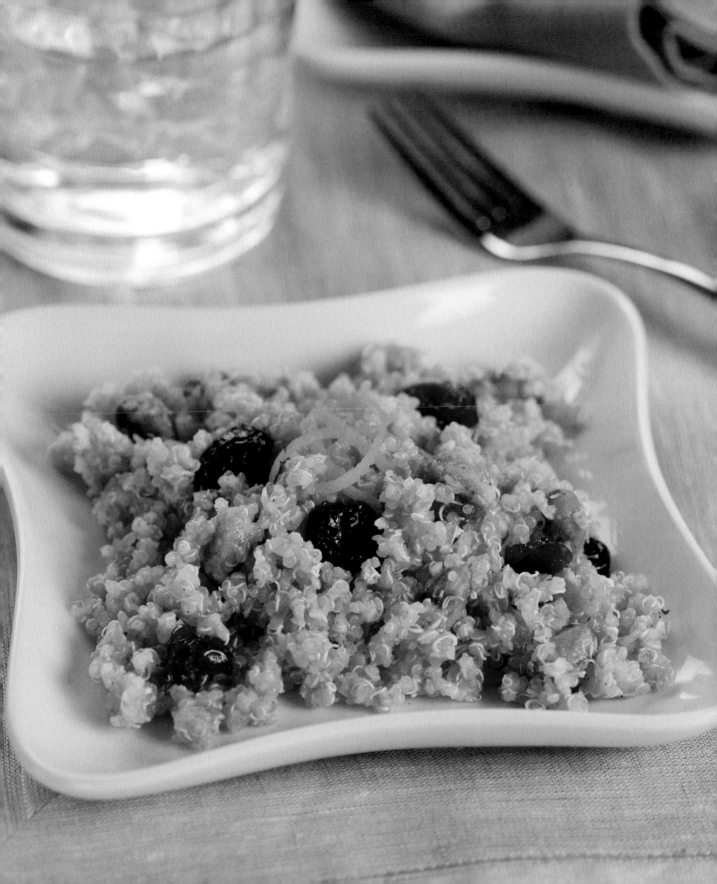

SWEET & SAVORY SWEET POTATO SALAD

MAKES 6 SERVINGS

4 cups peeled chopped cooked sweet potatoes (about 4 to 6)

¾ cup chopped green onions

½ cup chopped fresh parsley

½ cup dried unsweetened cherries

¼ cup plus 2 tablespoons rice wine vinegar

2 tablespoons coarse ground mustard

1 tablespoon extra virgin olive oil

¾ teaspoon garlic powder

¼ teaspoon black pepper

⅛ teaspoon salt

1. Combine sweet potatoes, green onions, parsley and cherries in large bowl; mix gently.

2. Whisk vinegar, mustard, oil, garlic powder, pepper and salt in small bowl until well blended. Pour over sweet potato mixture; toss gently to coat. Serve immediately or cover and refrigerate until ready to serve.

PER SERVING

CALORIES
161

TOTAL FAT
3g

SATURATED FAT
0g

CHOLESTEROL
0mg

SODIUM
116mg

CARBS
33g

DIETARY FIBER
4g

PROTEIN
3g

DIETARY EXCHANGES

2 bread/starch, ½ fat

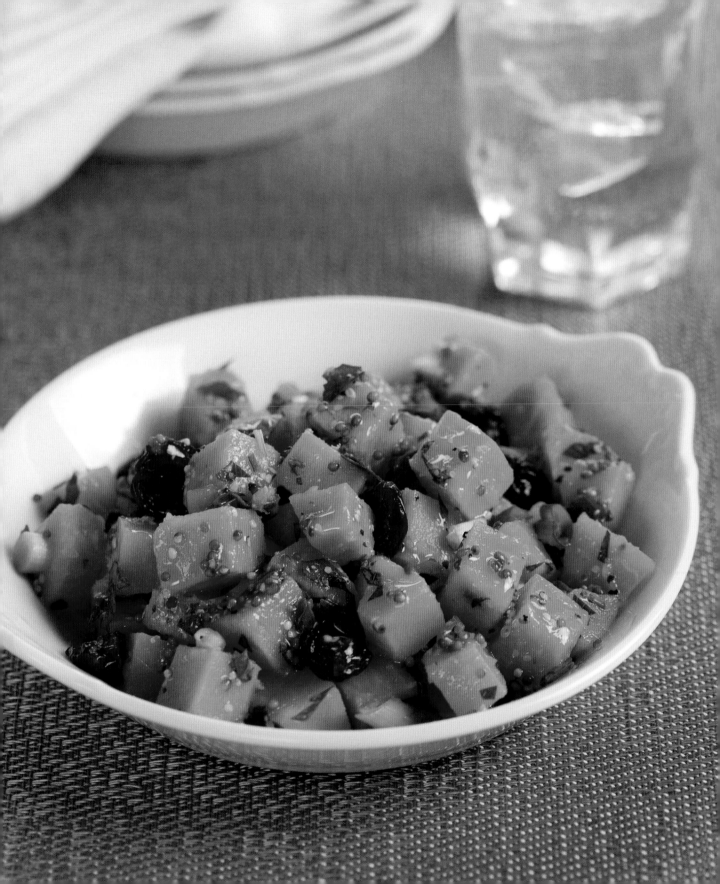

MASHED POTATO PUFFS

MAKES 18 PUFFS (ABOUT 6 SERVINGS)

1 **cup prepared mashed potatoes**

½ **cup finely chopped broccoli or spinach**

2 **egg whites**

4 **tablespoons shredded Parmesan cheese, divided**

1. Preheat oven to 400°F. Spray 18 mini (1¾-inch) muffin cups with nonstick cooking spray.

2. Combine mashed potatoes, broccoli, egg whites and 2 tablespoons Parmesan cheese in large bowl; mix well. Spoon evenly into prepared muffin cups. Sprinkle with remaining 2 tablespoons cheese.

3. Bake 20 to 23 minutes or until golden brown. To remove from pan, gently run knife around outer edges and lift out with fork. Serve warm.

PER SERVING

CALORIES
63

TOTAL FAT
2g

SATURATED FAT
1g

CHOLESTEROL
2mg

SODIUM
99mg

CARBS
8g

DIETARY FIBER
1g

PROTEIN
32g

DIETARY EXCHANGES

1 vegetable, ½ fat

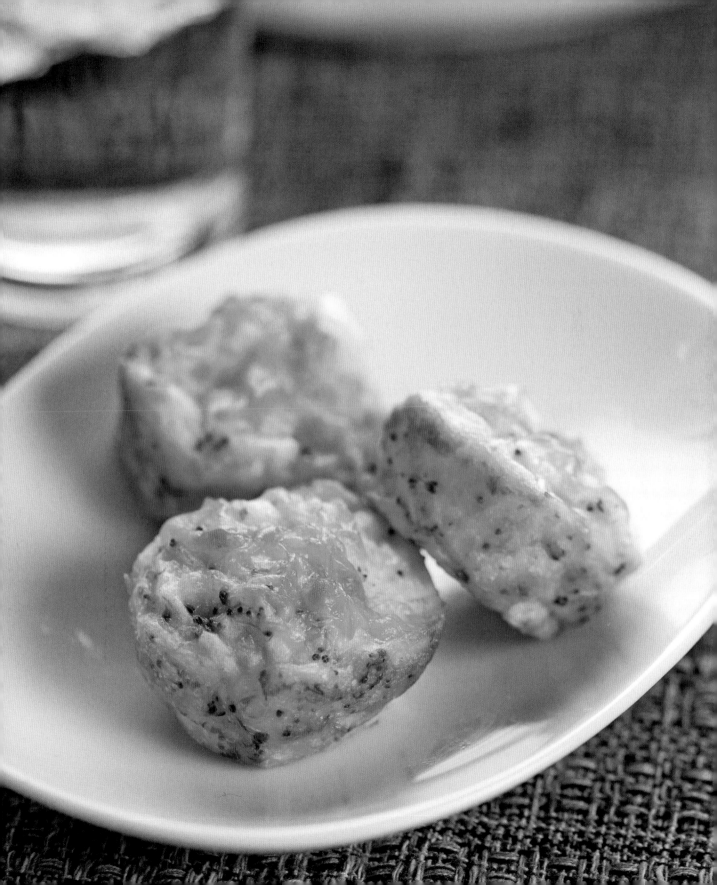

BUTTERNUT SQUASH OVEN FRIES

MAKES 4 SERVINGS

½ teaspoon garlic powder

¼ teaspoon salt

¼ teaspoon ground red pepper

1 butternut squash (about 2½ pounds), peeled, seeded and cut into 2-inch-thin slices

2 teaspoons vegetable oil

1. Preheat oven to 425°F. Combine garlic powder, salt and ground red pepper in small bowl; set aside.

2. Place squash on baking sheet. Drizzle with oil and sprinkle with seasoning mix; gently toss to coat. Arrange in single layer.

3. Bake 20 to 25 minutes or until squash just begins to brown, stirring frequently.

4. Preheat broiler. Broil 3 to 5 minutes or until fries are browned and crisp. Spread on paper towels to cool slightly before serving.

PER SERVING

CALORIES
129

TOTAL FAT
3g

SATURATED FAT
0g

CHOLESTEROL
0mg

SODIUM
155mg

CARBS
28g

DIETARY FIBER
5g

PROTEIN
2g

DIETARY EXCHANGES

1½ bread/starch, ½ fat

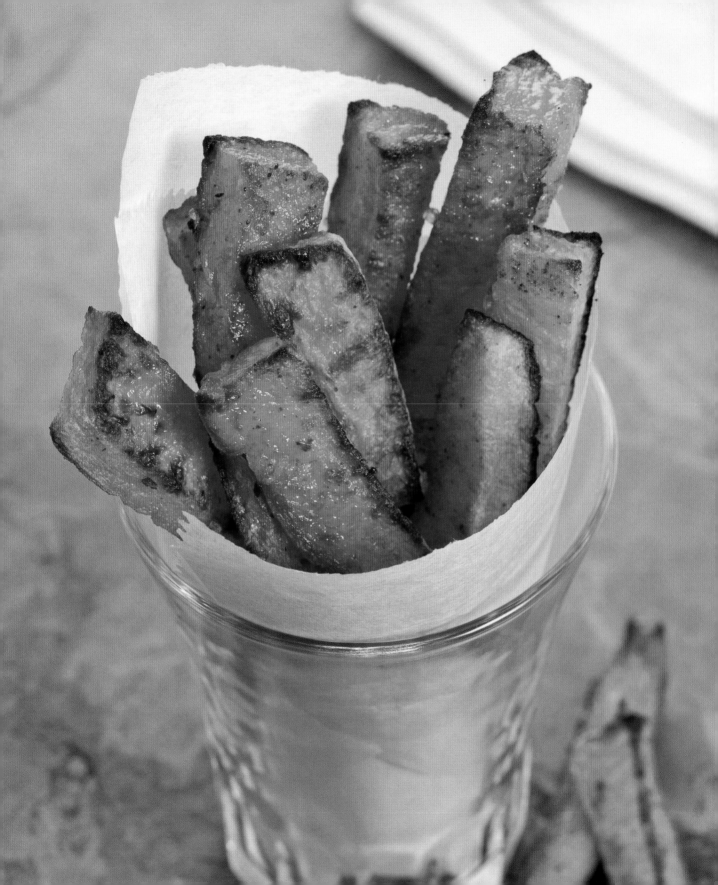

BROCCOLI SUPREME

MAKES 7 SERVINGS

2 packages (10 ounces each) frozen chopped broccoli

1 cup fat-free reduced-sodium chicken or vegetable broth

2 tablespoons reduced-fat mayonnaise

2 teaspoons dried minced onion (optional)

1. Combine broccoli, broth, mayonnaise and onion, if desired, in large saucepan. Cover and simmer over medium heat until broccoli is tender, stirring occasionally.

2. Uncover; continue to simmer until liquid has evaporated, stirring occasionally.

PER SERVING

CALORIES
31

TOTAL FAT
1g

SATURATED FAT
1g

CHOLESTEROL
1mg

SODIUM
26mg

CARBS
4g

DIETARY FIBER
2g

PROTEIN
2g

DIETARY EXCHANGES

1 vegetable

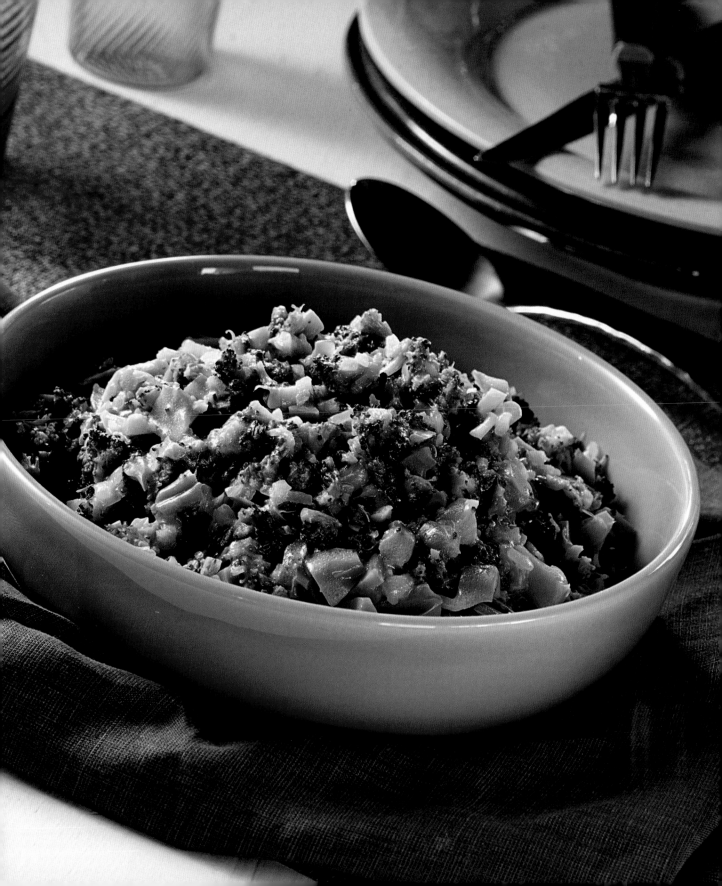

QUINOA & ROASTED VEGETABLES

MAKES 6 SERVINGS

- 2 medium sweet potatoes, cut into ½-inch-thick slices
- 1 medium eggplant, peeled and cut into ½-inch cubes
- 1 medium tomato, cut into wedges
- 1 large green bell pepper, sliced
- 1 small onion, cut into wedges
- ½ teaspoon salt
- ¼ teaspoon black pepper
- ¼ teaspoon ground red pepper
- 1 cup uncooked quinoa
- 2 cloves garlic, minced
- ½ teaspoon dried thyme
- ¼ teaspoon dried marjoram
- 2 cups water or fat-free reduced-sodium vegetable broth

1. Preheat oven to 450°F. Line large jelly-roll pan with foil; spray with nonstick cooking spray.

2. Combine sweet potatoes, eggplant, tomato, bell pepper and onion on prepared pan; spray lightly with cooking spray. Sprinkle with salt, black pepper and ground red pepper; toss to coat. Spread vegetables in single layer. Roast 20 to 30 minutes or until vegetables are browned and tender.

3. Meanwhile, place quinoa in fine-mesh strainer; rinse well under cold running water. Spray medium saucepan with cooking spray; heat over medium heat. Add garlic, thyme and marjoram; cook and stir 1 to 2 minutes. Add quinoa; cook and stir 2 to 3 minutes. Stir in 2 cups water; bring to a boil over high heat. Reduce heat to low. Simmer, covered, 15 to 20 minutes or until water is absorbed. (Quinoa will appear somewhat translucent.) Transfer quinoa to large bowl; gently stir in roasted vegetables.

PER SERVING

CALORIES
193

TOTAL FAT
2g

SATURATED FAT
1g

CHOLESTEROL
0mg

SODIUM
194mg

CARBS
40g

DIETARY FIBER
6g

PROTEIN
6g

DIETARY EXCHANGES

2½ bread/starch, ½ vegetable

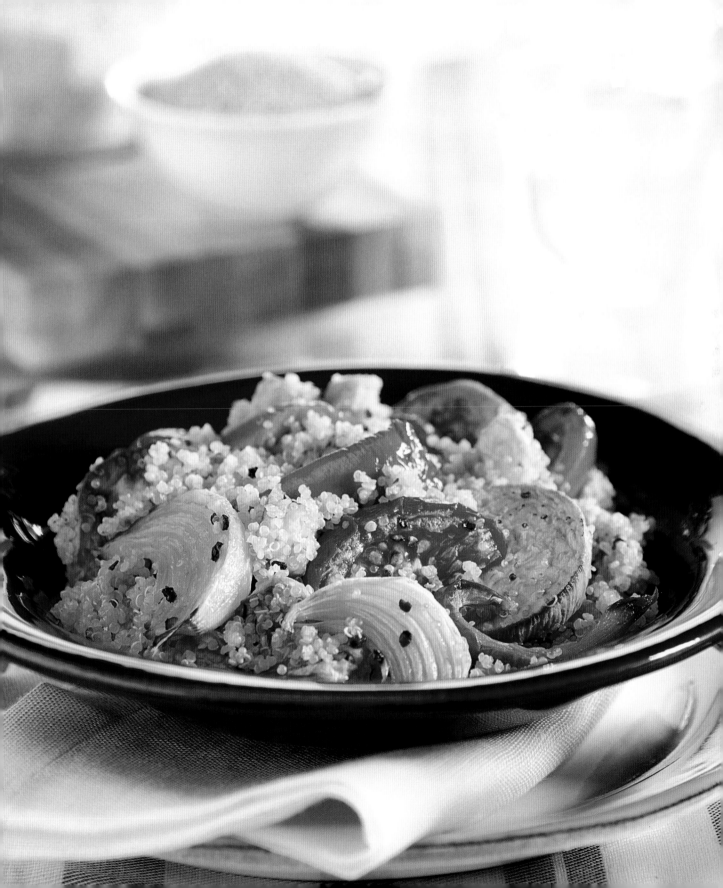

SWEET POTATO BISCUITS

MAKES 12 BISCUITS

1½ cups all-purpose flour, plus additional for work surface

2 tablespoons packed dark brown sugar

1 tablespoon baking powder

½ teaspoon salt

½ teaspoon ground cinnamon

⅛ teaspoon ground nutmeg

5 tablespoons unsalted butter, cut into small pieces

1 cold puréed cooked sweet potato (about 1 large sweet potato)

½ cup low-fat buttermilk

2 tablespoons honey

1. Preheat oven to 450°F. Spray baking sheet with nonstick cooking spray.

2. Combine 1½ cups flour, brown sugar, baking powder, salt, cinnamon and nutmeg in medium bowl; mix well. Cut in butter with pastry blender or two knives until coarse crumbs form. Stir in sweet potato and buttermilk until combined.

3. Transfer dough to floured work surface. Using floured hands, knead dough five times or until no longer sticky, adding additional flour if necessary. Pat dough into ¼-inch-thick disc. Cut out dough with 2½-inch round biscuit cutter. Reroll scraps and cut out additional pieces. Place 1 inch apart on prepared baking sheet. Refrigerate 20 minutes.

4. Bake 12 to 14 minutes or until biscuits are light golden brown and puffed. Immediately brush tops evenly with honey. Remove to wire racks; cool 5 minutes. Serve warm.

PER SERVING

CALORIES
145

TOTAL FAT
5g

SATURATED FAT
3g

CHOLESTEROL
13mg

SODIUM
239mg

CARBS
23g

DIETARY FIBER
1g

PROTEIN
2g

DIETARY EXCHANGES

1½ bread/starch, 1 fat

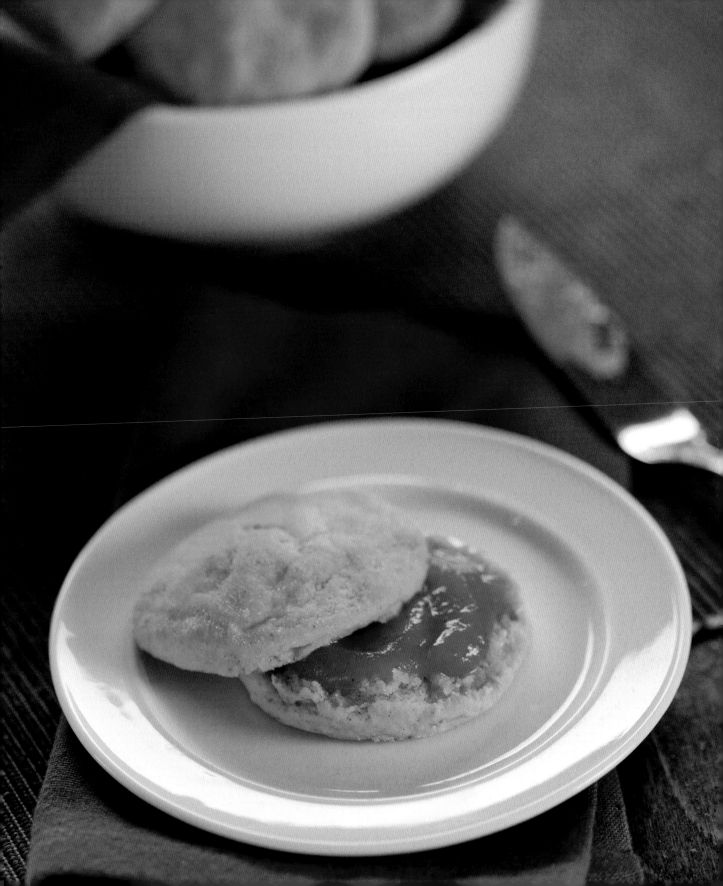

GINGER NOODLES WITH SESAME EGG STRIPS

MAKES 4 SERVINGS

5 **egg whites**

6 **teaspoons teriyaki sauce, divided**

3 **teaspoons sesame seeds, toasted,* divided**

1 **teaspoon dark sesame oil**

½ **cup fat-free reduced-sodium chicken broth**

1 **tablespoon minced fresh ginger**

6 **ounces Chinese rice noodles or vermicelli noodles, cooked and well drained**

⅓ **cup sliced green onions**

*To toast sesame seeds, spread in small skillet. Shake skillet over medium-low heat 3 minutes or until seeds begin to pop and turn golden.

1. Beat egg whites, 2 teaspoons teriyaki sauce and 1 teaspoon sesame seeds in medium bowl until well blended.

2. Heat oil in large nonstick skillet over medium heat. Pour in egg mixture; cook 1½ to 2 minutes or until bottom is set. Turn over; cook 30 seconds to 1 minute or until cooked through. Gently slide onto plate; cut into ½-inch strips when cool enough to handle.

3. Add broth, ginger and remaining 4 teaspoons teriyaki sauce to skillet; bring to a boil over high heat. Reduce heat to medium; stir in noodles. Cook until heated through. Add omelet strips and green onions; heat through. Sprinkle with remaining 2 teaspoons sesame seeds just before serving.

PER SERVING

CALORIES
210

TOTAL FAT
3g

SATURATED FAT
0g

CHOLESTEROL
0mg

SODIUM
300mg

CARBS
38g

DIETARY FIBER
1g

PROTEIN
8g

DIETARY EXCHANGES

2 bread/starch, ½ fat

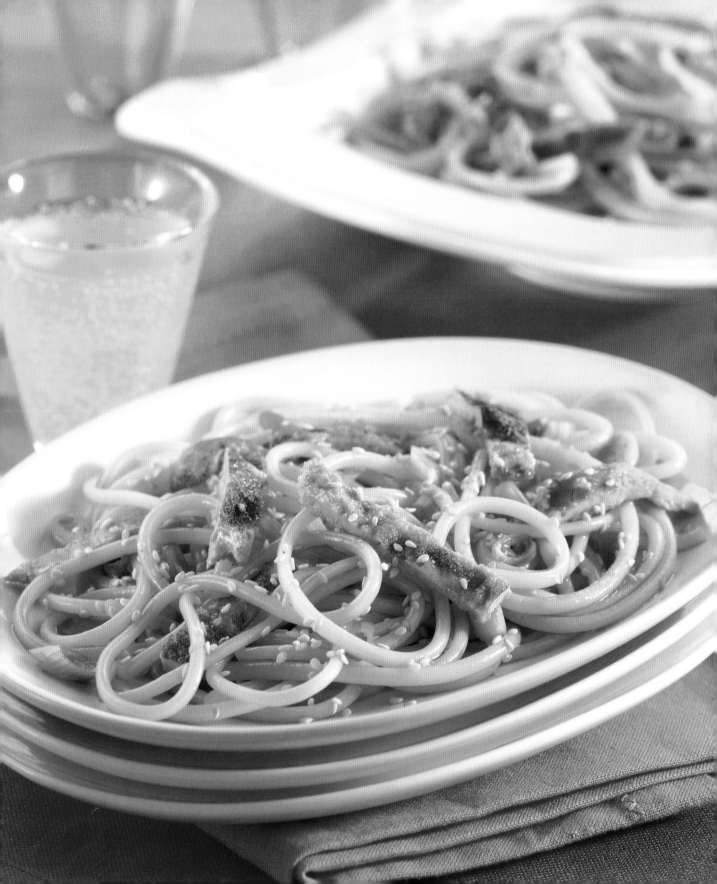

TABBOULEH IN TOMATO CUPS

MAKES 8 SERVINGS

4 large firm ripe tomatoes (about 8 ounces each)

2 tablespoons olive oil

4 green onions with tops, thinly sliced diagonally, divided

1 cup uncooked bulgur wheat

1 cup water

2 tablespoons lemon juice

1 tablespoon chopped fresh mint leaves *or* ½ teaspoon dried mint

Salt and black pepper

Lemon peel and fresh mint leaves (optional)

1. Cut tomatoes in half crosswise. Scoop pulp and seeds out of tomatoes into medium bowl, leaving ¼-inch-thick shells.

2. Invert tomatoes on paper towel-lined plate; drain 20 minutes. Chop tomato pulp; set aside.

3. Heat oil in medium saucepan over medium-high heat. Cook and stir white parts of green onions 1 to 2 minutes or until wilted. Add bulgur; cook 3 to 5 minutes or until browned.

4. Add reserved tomato pulp, water, lemon juice and 1 tablespoon chopped mint to bulgur mixture. Bring to a boil over high heat; reduce heat to medium-low. Cover; simmer gently 15 to 20 minutes or until liquid is absorbed.

5. Set aside a few sliced green onions for garnish; stir remaining green onions into bulgur mixture. Season with salt and pepper. Spoon mixture into tomato cups.*

6. Preheat oven to 400°F. Place filled cups in 13×9-inch baking dish; bake 15 minutes or until heated through. Top with reserved onion tops. Garnish with lemon peel and mint leaves. Serve immediately.

Tomato cups may be covered and refrigerated at this point up to 24 hours.

PER SERVING

CALORIES
210

TOTAL FAT
8g

SATURATED FAT
1g

CHOLESTEROL
0mg

SODIUM
15mg

CARBS
34g

DIETARY FIBER
8g

PROTEIN
6g

DIETARY EXCHANGES

2 bread/starch, 1½ fat

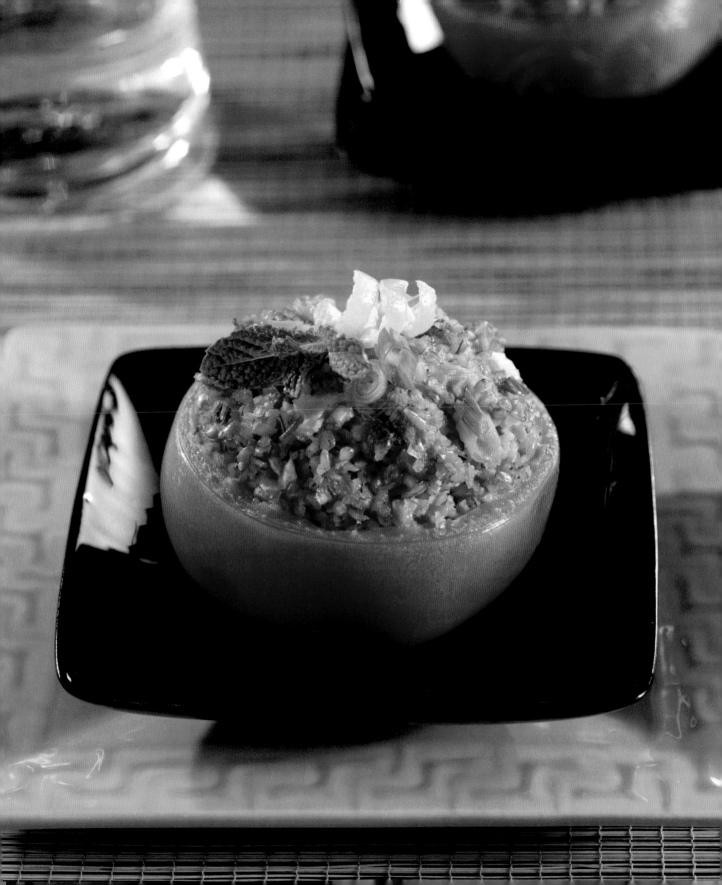

SZECHUAN EGGPLANT

MAKES 4 SERVINGS

1 **pound Asian eggplants or regular eggplant, peeled**

2 **tablespoons peanut or vegetable oil**

2 **cloves garlic, minced**

¼ **teaspoon red pepper flakes** *or* ½ **teaspoon hot chili oil**

¼ **cup vegetable broth**

¼ **cup hoisin sauce**

3 **green onions, cut into 1-inch pieces**

Toasted sesame seeds* (optional)

*To toast sesame seeds, spread in small skillet. Shake skillet over medium-low heat 3 minutes or until seeds begin to pop and turn golden.

1. Cut eggplants into ½-inch slices; cut each slice into ½×½-inch strips.

2. Heat wok or large nonstick skillet over medium-high heat. Add peanut oil; heat until hot. Add eggplant, garlic and red pepper flakes; stir-fry 7 minutes or until eggplant is very tender and browned.

3. Reduce heat to medium. Add broth, hoisin sauce and green onions to wok; cook and stir 2 minutes. Sprinkle with sesame seeds, if desired.

PER SERVING

CALORIES
130

TOTAL FAT
8g

SATURATED FAT
1.5g

CHOLESTEROL
0mg

SODIUM
290mg

CARBS
14g

DIETARY FIBER
3g

PROTEIN
2g

DIETARY EXCHANGES

1 bread/starch, 1½ fat

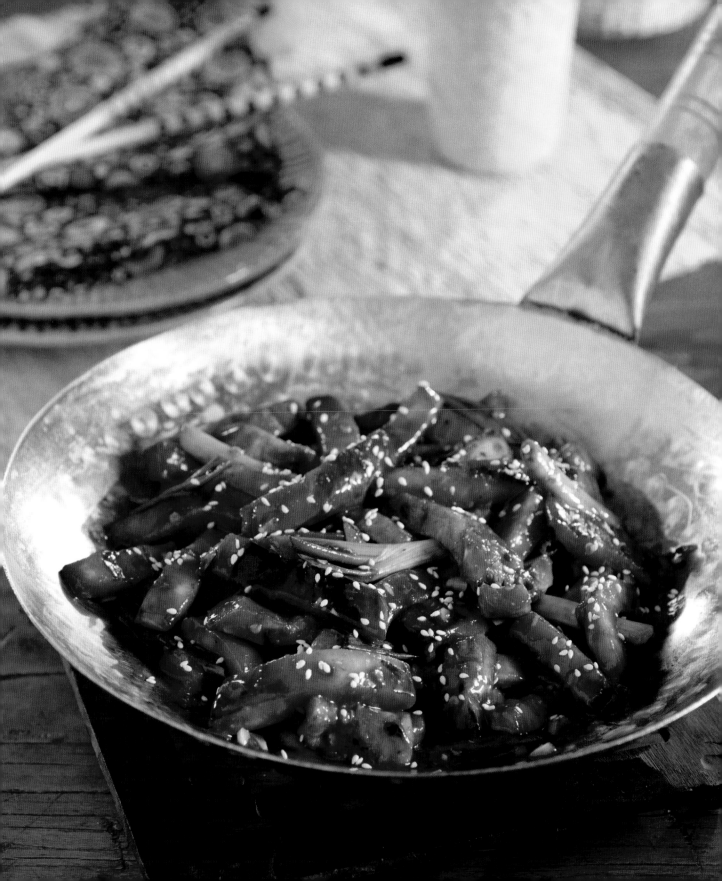

MEDITERRANEAN ORZO AND VEGETABLE PILAF

MAKES 6 SERVINGS

- 4 ounces (½ cup plus 2 tablespoons) uncooked orzo pasta
- 2 teaspoons olive oil
- 1 small onion, diced
- 2 cloves garlic, minced
- 1 small zucchini, diced
- ½ cup fat-free reduced-sodium chicken broth
- 1 can (about 14 ounces) artichoke hearts, drained and quartered
- 1 medium tomato, chopped
- ½ teaspoon dried oregano
- ½ teaspoon salt
- ¼ teaspoon black pepper
- ½ cup (2 ounces) crumbled feta cheese
- Sliced black olives (optional)

1. Cook orzo according to package directions, omitting salt and fat. Drain.

2. Heat oil in large nonstick skillet over medium heat. Add onion; cook and stir 5 minutes or until translucent. Add garlic; cook and stir 1 minute. Reduce heat to low. Add zucchini and broth; simmer 5 minutes or until zucchini is crisp-tender.

3. Add cooked orzo, artichokes, tomato, oregano, salt and pepper; cook and stir 1 minute or until heated through. Top with feta cheese and olives, if desired.

Note

This makes a nice side dish to any plain grilled or roasted chicken or fish.

Tip

To reduce the sodium in this recipe, omit the salt. With all the different fresh flavors, you will not miss the extra salt.

PER SERVING

CALORIES
170

TOTAL FAT
4g

SATURATED FAT
1.5g

CHOLESTEROL
10mg

SODIUM
720mg

CARBS
25g

DIETARY FIBER
2g

PROTEIN
7g

DIETARY EXCHANGES

1 bread/starch, 2 vegetable, ½ fat

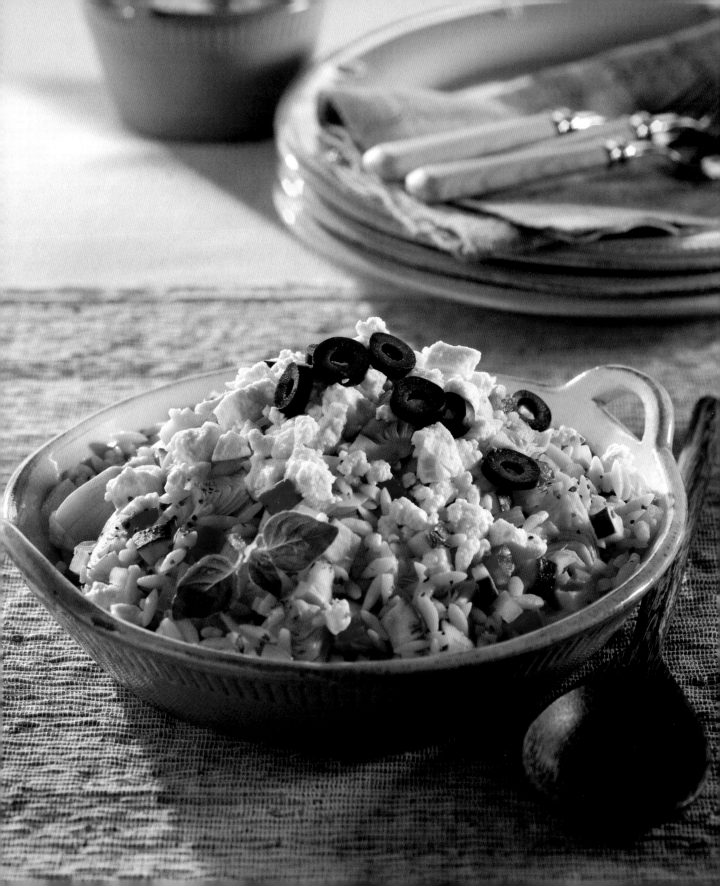

OLD-FASHIONED HERB STUFFING

MAKES 4 SERVINGS

6 slices (8 ounces) whole wheat, rye or white bread (or combination), cut into ½-inch cubes

1 tablespoon margarine or butter

1 cup chopped onion

½ cup thinly sliced celery

½ cup thinly sliced carrot

1 cup fat-free reduced-sodium chicken broth

1 tablespoon chopped fresh thyme *or* 1 teaspoon dried thyme

1 tablespoon chopped fresh sage *or* 1 teaspoon dried sage

½ teaspoon paprika

¼ teaspoon black pepper

1. Preheat oven to 350°F. Spray 1½-quart baking dish with nonstick cooking spray.

2. Place bread cubes on baking sheet; bake 10 minutes or until dry.

3. Melt margarine in large saucepan over medium heat. Add onion, celery and carrot; cook and stir 10 minutes or until vegetables are tender. Add broth, thyme, sage, paprika and pepper; bring to a simmer. Stir in bread cubes. Spoon into prepared baking dish.

4. Cover and bake 25 to 30 minutes or until heated through.

PER SERVING

CALORIES
199

TOTAL FAT
5g

SATURATED FAT
1g

CHOLESTEROL
0mg

SODIUM
395mg

CARBS
32g

DIETARY FIBER
5g

PROTEIN
8g

DIETARY EXCHANGES

2 bread/starch, 1 fat

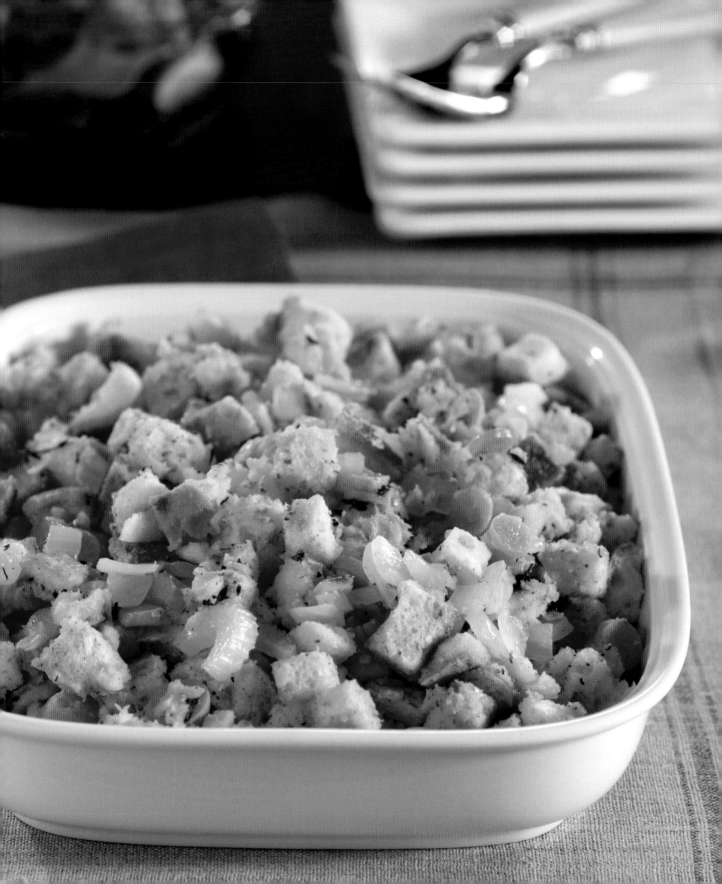

MASHED SWEET POTATOES & PARSNIPS

MAKES 6 SERVINGS

2 large sweet potatoes (about 1¼ pounds), peeled and cut into 1-inch pieces

2 medium parsnips (about ½ pound), peeled and cut into ½-inch slices

¼ cup evaporated skimmed milk

1½ tablespoons butter or margarine

½ teaspoon salt

⅛ teaspoon ground nutmeg

¼ cup chopped fresh chives or green onions

1. Combine sweet potatoes and parsnips in large saucepan. Cover with cold water; bring to a boil over high heat. Reduce heat; simmer, uncovered, 15 minutes or until vegetables are tender.

2. Drain vegetables; return to pan. Add milk, butter, salt and nutmeg. Mash with potato masher over low heat until desired consistency is reached. Stir in chives.

PER SERVING

CALORIES
136

TOTAL FAT
3g

SATURATED FAT
2g

CHOLESTEROL
8mg

SODIUM
243mg

CARBS
25g

DIETARY FIBER
5g

PROTEIN
3g

DIETARY EXCHANGES

1½ bread/starch, ½ fat

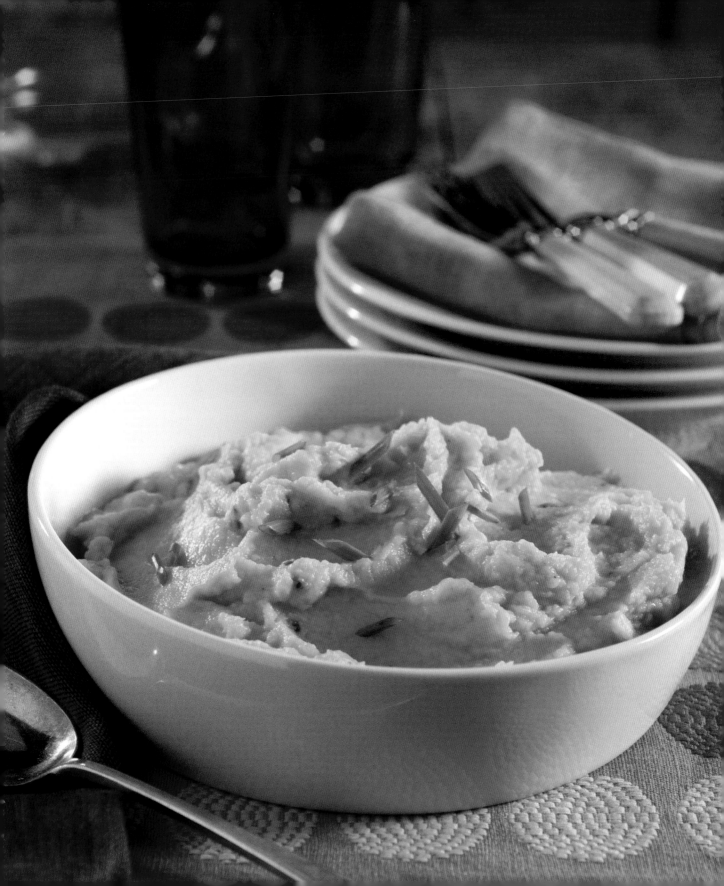

PEPPER AND SQUASH GRATIN

- 1 russet potato, unpeeled
- 1 medium yellow summer squash, thinly sliced
- 1 medium zucchini, thinly sliced
- 2 cups frozen bell pepper stir-fry blend, thawed
- 1 teaspoon dried oregano
- ½ teaspoon salt
- ⅛ teaspoon black pepper (optional)
- ½ cup grated Parmesan cheese or shredded reduced-fat sharp Cheddar cheese
- 1 tablespoon butter or margarine, cut into 8 pieces

1. Preheat oven to 375°F. Spray 12×8-inch glass baking dish with nonstick cooking spray. Pierce potato several times with fork. Microwave on HIGH 3 minutes. Cut potato into thin slices.

2. Layer half of potato slices, yellow squash, zucchini, bell pepper stir-fry blend, oregano, salt, black pepper, if desired, and Parmesan cheese in prepared baking dish. Repeat layers. Dot with butter. Cover tightly with foil; bake 25 minutes or until vegetables are just tender. Remove foil; bake 10 minutes or until lightly browned.

PER SERVING

CALORIES
110

TOTAL FAT
5g

SATURATED FAT
3g

CHOLESTEROL
15mg

SODIUM
360mg

CARBS
11g

DIETARY FIBER
1g

PROTEIN
6g

DIETARY EXCHANGES

½ bread/starch,
½ meat,
½ vegetable,
1 fat

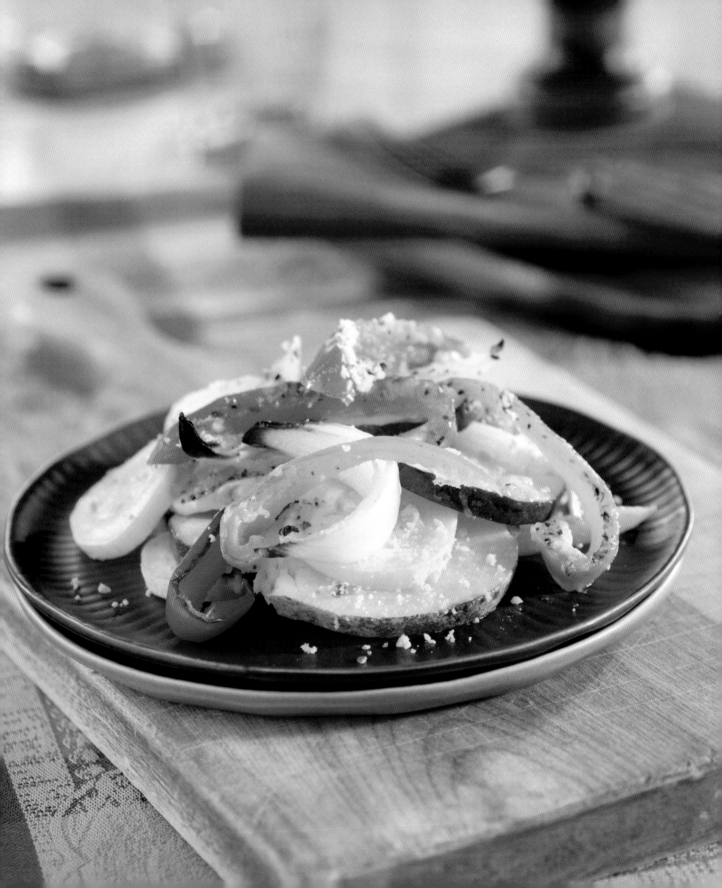

HERBED CAULIFLOWER CASSEROLE

MAKES 5 SERVINGS

- 5 cups cauliflower florets (about 1¼ pounds)
- 1 tablespoon reduced-fat margarine, melted
- 1 small red bell pepper, cut into quarters
- 2 tablespoons water
- 3 large tomatoes, peeled, seeded and coarsely chopped
- 2 to 3 teaspoons chopped fresh tarragon
- ½ teaspoon chopped fresh parsley
- ⅓ cup (9 to 10) coarsely crushed unsalted saltine crackers

1. Preheat oven to 450°F.

2. Toss cauliflower with margarine in large bowl; place cauliflower and bell pepper, cut sides down, in single layer in shallow baking pan. Add water to pan.

3. Bake 15 minutes. *Reduce oven temperature to 425°F.*

4. Bake 25 to 28 minutes or until cauliflower is tender and golden brown and bell pepper skin is blistered. Remove bell pepper pieces to plate and transfer cauliflower to 11×7-inch baking dish. *Reduce oven temperature to 400°F.*

5. Remove and discard skin from bell pepper. Place tomatoes and bell pepper in food processor; process until smooth. Add tarragon and parsley; process until blended. Pour tomato sauce over cauliflower.

6. Bake 10 minutes or until hot and bubbly. Sprinkle with cracker crumbs just before serving.

PER SERVING

CALORIES
80

TOTAL FAT
2g

SATURATED FAT
1g

CHOLESTEROL
0mg

SODIUM
100mg

CARBS
14g

DIETARY FIBER
4g

PROTEIN
3g

DIETARY EXCHANGES

2½ vegetable, ½ fat

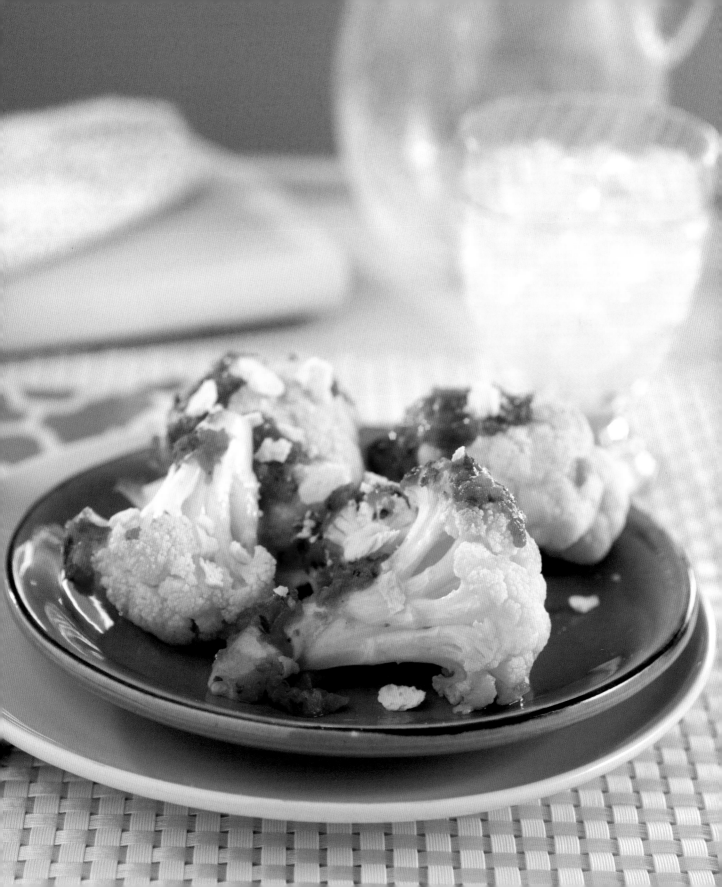

SPINACH AND MUSHROOM RISOTTO

MAKES 8 SERVINGS

½ **pound mushrooms, sliced**

2 **teaspoons dried basil**

2 **teaspoons minced garlic**

¼ **teaspoon black pepper**

1 **can (about 14 ounces) fat-free reduced-sodium chicken broth**

1⅔ **cups water**

1½ **cups uncooked arborio rice**

1 **can (about 10¾ ounces) reduced-fat reduced-sodium condensed cream of mushroom soup, undiluted**

3 **cups packed stemmed spinach, chopped**

6 **tablespoons chopped walnuts, toasted***

¼ **cup grated Parmesan cheese**

*To toast walnuts, cook in small skillet over medium heat 6 to 8 minutes or until fragrant, stirring frequently.

1. Coat 3-quart saucepan with olive oil nonstick cooking spray. Cook and stir mushrooms, basil, garlic and pepper over high heat 3 to 4 minutes or until mushrooms are tender.

2. Add broth, water, rice and soup; cook and stir until well blended and mixture begins to boil. Reduce heat to low. Cover; simmer gently 12 minutes, stirring twice during cooking, or until rice is just tender but still firm.

3. Stir in spinach; cover and let stand 5 to 7 minutes or until spinach is wilted.

4. Sprinkle with walnuts and Parmesan cheese before serving.

PER SERVING

CALORIES
219

TOTAL FAT
5g

SATURATED FAT
1g

CHOLESTEROL
2mg

SODIUM
250mg

CARBS
37g

DIETARY FIBER
3g

PROTEIN
8g

DIETARY EXCHANGES

1½ bread/starch, 2 vegetable, 1 fat

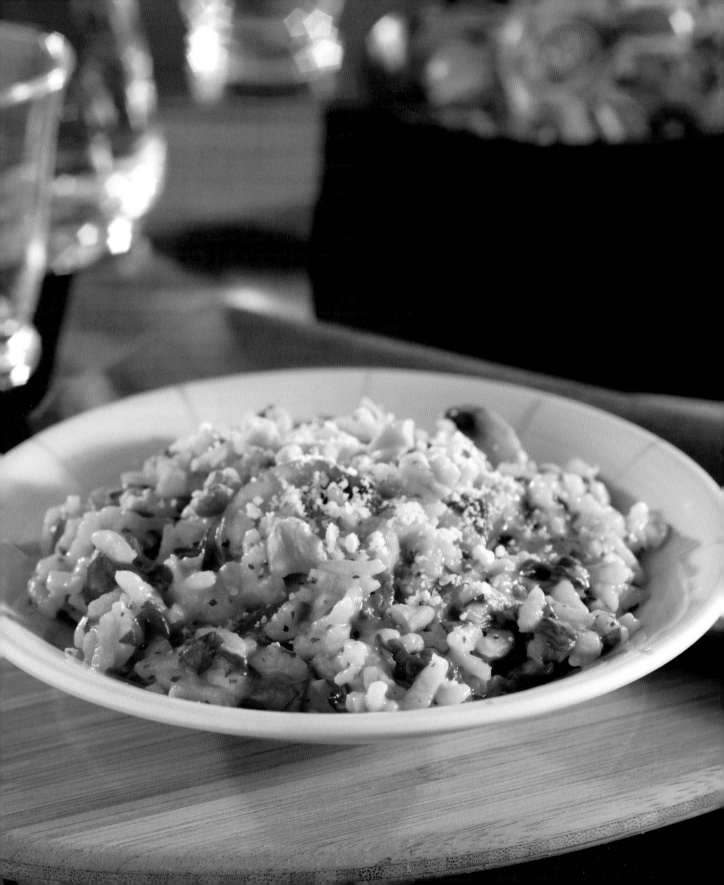

PASTA PRIMAVERA

MAKES 4 SERVINGS

- 8 ounces uncooked linguine
- 1 tablespoon reduced-fat margarine
- 2 green onions, sliced diagonally
- 1 clove garlic, minced
- 1 cup mushroom slices
- 1 cup broccoli florets
- 2½ cups fresh snow peas
- 4 asparagus spears, cut into 2-inch pieces
- 1 red bell pepper, cut into thin strips
- ½ cup evaporated skimmed milk
- ½ teaspoon dried tarragon leaves
- ½ teaspoon black pepper
- ⅓ cup grated Parmesan cheese

1. Cook pasta according to package directions, omitting salt. Drain; set aside.

2. Melt margarine in large nonstick skillet. Add green onions and garlic; cook over medium heat until softened. Add mushrooms and broccoli. Cover; cook 3 minutes or until mushrooms are tender. Add snow peas, asparagus, bell pepper, milk, tarragon and black pepper. Cook and stir until vegetables are crisp-tender and lightly coated.

3. Add Parmesan cheese and linguine; toss to coat.

PER SERVING

CALORIES
337

TOTAL FAT
7g

SATURATED FAT
3g

CHOLESTEROL
10mg

SODIUM
244mg

CARBS
54g

DIETARY FIBER
5g

PROTEIN
17g

DIETARY EXCHANGES

3 bread/starch,
½ meat,
1½ vegetable,
½ fat

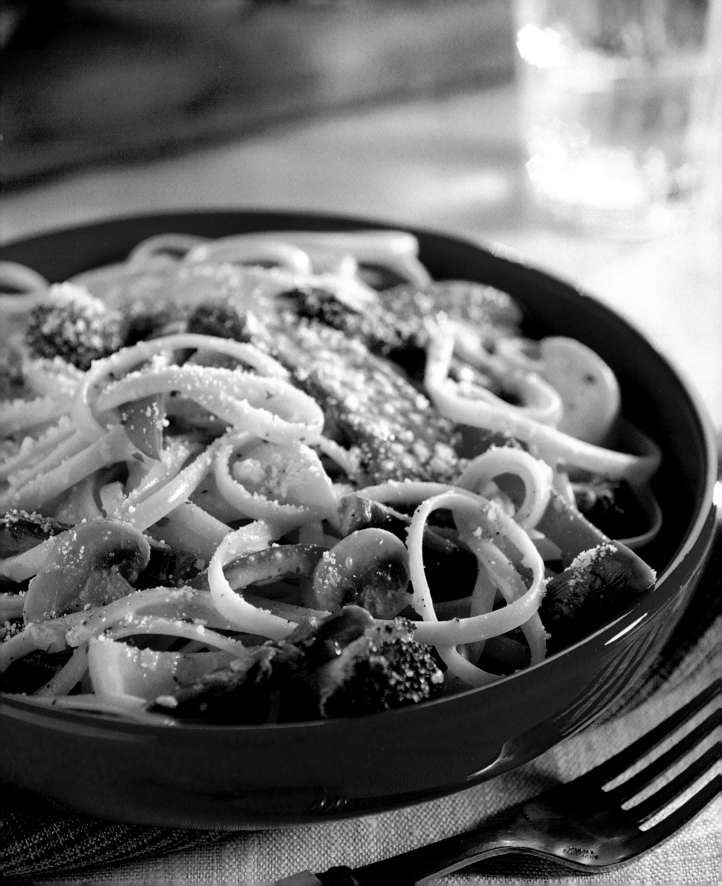

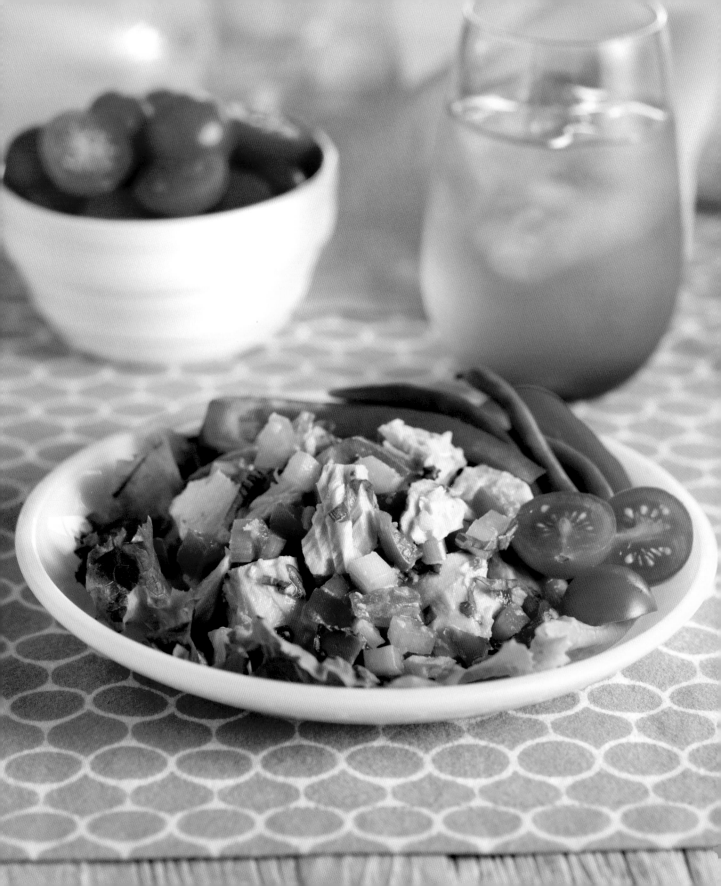

HEARTY & SIDE SALADS

MEDITERRANEAN TUNA SALAD

MAKES 4 SERVINGS

1 cup diced tomato

1 tablespoon olive oil

1 tablespoon lemon juice

2 teaspoons Dijon mustard

1 clove garlic, minced

¼ teaspoon salt

¼ teaspoon dried basil

2 cans (5 ounces each) solid white tuna packed in water, drained and flaked

½ cup diced celery

⅓ cup chopped fresh basil

Red leaf lettuce leaves

½ pound steamed green beans

1 medium red bell pepper, cut into strips

8 cherry tomatoes, halved

1. Combine diced tomato, oil, lemon juice, mustard, garlic, salt and dried basil in large bowl; let stand 5 minutes. Stir in tuna, celery and fresh basil. Refrigerate, covered, 1 to 2 hours to allow flavors to blend, stirring once.

2. Line serving platter with lettuce leaves. Mound tuna salad in center; serve with green beans, bell pepper and cherry tomatoes.

PER SERVING

CALORIES
170

TOTAL FAT
6g

SATURATED FAT
1g

CHOLESTEROL
30mg

SODIUM
490mg

CARBS
9g

DIETARY FIBER
3g

PROTEIN
19g

DIETARY EXCHANGES

2 meat,
2 vegetable,
½ fat

CRAB SPINACH SALAD WITH TARRAGON DRESSING

MAKES 4 SERVINGS

12 ounces coarsely flaked cooked crabmeat *or* 2 packages (6 ounces each) frozen crabmeat, thawed and drained

1 cup chopped tomatoes

1 cup sliced cucumber

⅓ cup sliced red onion

¼ cup fat-free salad dressing or mayonnaise

¼ cup reduced-fat sour cream

¼ cup chopped fresh parsley

2 tablespoons fat-free (skim) milk

2 teaspoons chopped fresh tarragon *or* ½ teaspoon dried tarragon leaves

1 clove garlic, minced

¼ teaspoon hot pepper sauce

8 cups fresh spinach

1. Combine crabmeat, tomatoes, cucumber and onion in medium bowl. Combine salad dressing, sour cream, parsley, milk, tarragon, garlic and hot pepper sauce in small bowl.

2. Line 4 salad plates with spinach. Place crabmeat mixture on spinach; drizzle with dressing.

PER SERVING

CALORIES
170

TOTAL FAT
4g

SATURATED FAT
1g

CHOLESTEROL
91mg

SODIUM
481mg

CARBS
14g

DIETARY FIBER
4g

PROTEIN
22g

DIETARY EXCHANGES

2 vegetable, 2½ meat

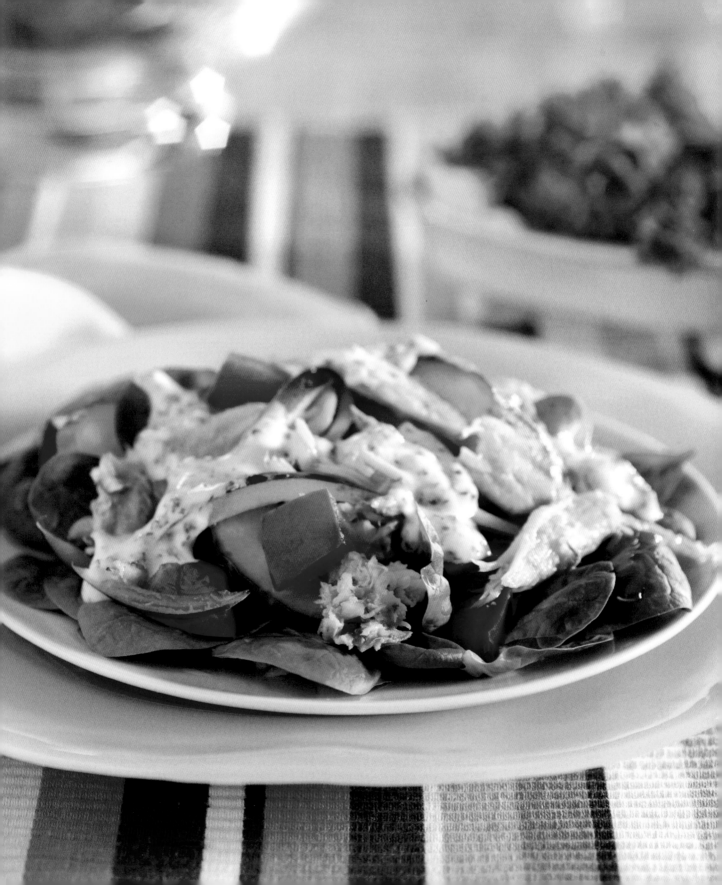

COLD PEANUT NOODLE AND EDAMAME SALAD

MAKES 4 SERVINGS

- ½ of an 8-ounce package brown rice pad thai noodles
- 3 tablespoons soy sauce
- 2 tablespoons dark sesame oil
- 2 tablespoons unseasoned rice vinegar
- 1 tablespoon sugar
- 1 tablespoon finely grated fresh ginger
- 1 tablespoon creamy peanut butter
- 1 tablespoon sriracha or hot chili sauce
- 2 teaspoons minced garlic
- ½ cup thawed frozen shelled edamame
- ¼ cup shredded carrots
- ¼ cup sliced green onions
- Chopped peanuts (optional)

1. Prepare noodles according to package directions for pasta. Rinse under cold water; drain. Cut noodles into 3-inch lengths. Place in large bowl; set aside.

2. Whisk soy sauce, oil, vinegar, sugar, ginger, peanut butter, sriracha and garlic in small bowl until smooth and well blended.

3. Pour dressing over noodles; toss gently to coat. Stir in edamame and carrots. Cover and refrigerate at least 30 minutes before serving. Top with green onions and peanuts, if desired.

Note

Brown rice pad thai noodles can be found in the Asian section of the supermarket. Regular thin rice noodles or whole wheat spaghetti may be substituted.

PER SERVING

CALORIES
239

TOTAL FAT
10g

SATURATED FAT
1g

CHOLESTEROL
0mg

SODIUM
556mg

CARBS
32g

DIETARY FIBER
1g

PROTEIN
6g

DIETARY EXCHANGES

1½ bread/starch,
1 vegetable,
2 fat

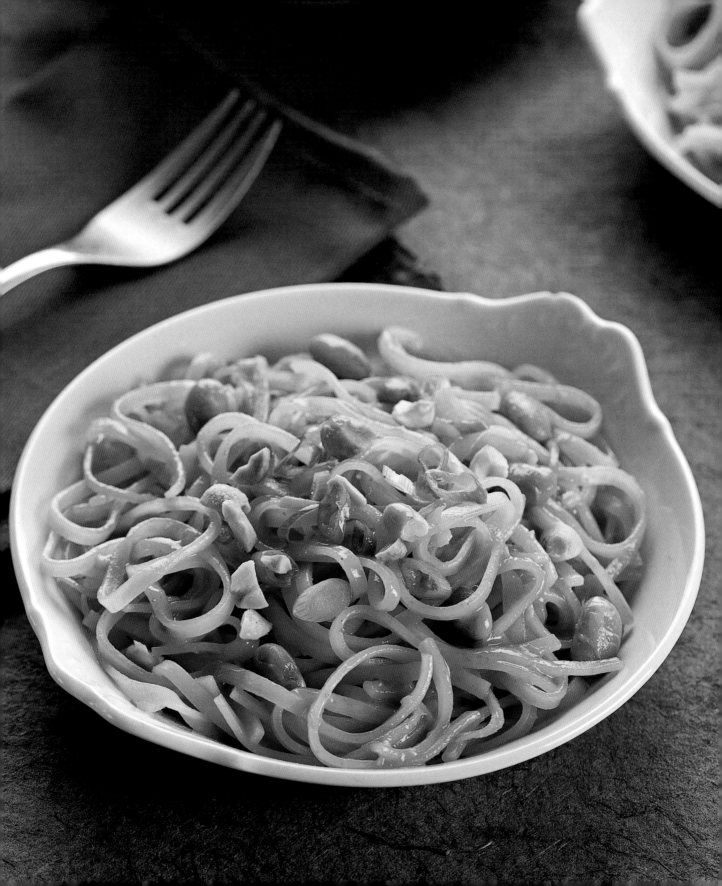

GRILLED STONE FRUIT SALAD

MAKES 4 SERVINGS

- 2 tablespoons fresh orange juice
- 1 tablespoon fresh lemon juice
- 2 teaspoons canola oil
- 1 teaspoon honey
- ½ teaspoon Dijon mustard
- 1 tablespoon finely chopped fresh mint
- 1 medium peach, halved and pit removed
- 1 medium nectarine, halved and pit removed
- 1 medium plum, halved and pit removed
- 4 cups mixed baby greens
- ½ cup crumbled goat cheese

1. Prepare grill for direct cooking over medium-high heat. Spray grid with nonstick cooking spray.

2. Whisk orange juice, lemon juice, oil, honey and mustard in small bowl until smooth and well blended. Stir in mint.

3. Brush cut sides of fruits with orange juice mixture. Set remaining dressing aside. Place fruits, cut sides down, on prepared grid. Grill, covered, 2 to 3 minutes. Turn over; grill 2 to 3 minutes or until fruits begin to soften. Remove to plate; let stand to cool slightly. When cool enough to handle, cut into wedges.

4. Arrange mixed greens on 4 serving plates. Top evenly with fruits and goat cheese. Drizzle with remaining dressing. Serve immediately.

PER SERVING

CALORIES
119

TOTAL FAT
6g

SATURATED FAT
3g

CHOLESTEROL
11mg

SODIUM
91mg

CARBS
14g

DIETARY FIBER
2g

PROTEIN
4g

DIETARY EXCHANGES

1 fruit,
1 fat

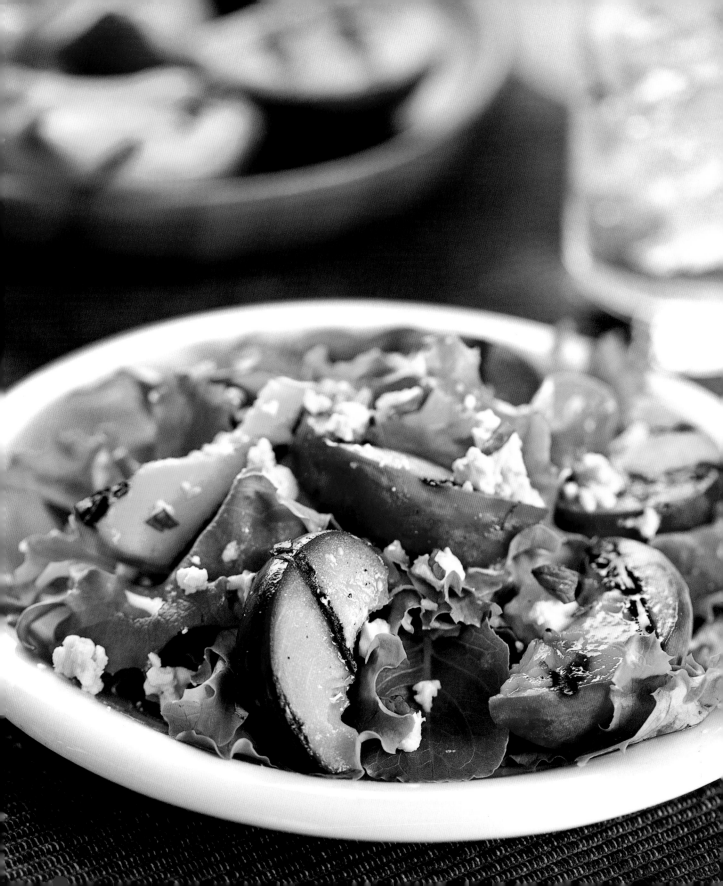

HEIRLOOM TOMATO QUINOA SALAD

MAKES 4 SERVINGS

1 cup uncooked quinoa

2 cups water

2 tablespoons olive oil

1 tablespoon lemon juice

1 clove garlic, minced

½ teaspoon salt

2 cups assorted heirloom grape tomatoes (red, yellow or a combination), halved

¼ cup crumbled fat-free feta cheese

¼ cup chopped fresh basil, plus additional basil leaves for garnish

1. Place quinoa in fine-mesh strainer; rinse well under cold running water. Bring 2 cups water to a boil in small saucepan; stir in quinoa. Reduce heat to low; cover and simmer 10 to 15 minutes or until quinoa is tender and water is absorbed.

2. Meanwhile, whisk oil, lemon juice, garlic and salt in large bowl until well blended. Gently stir in tomatoes and quinoa. Cover; refrigerate at least 30 minutes.

3. Stir in feta cheese just before serving. Top each serving with 1 tablespoon chopped basil. Garnish with additional basil leaves.

PER SERVING

CALORIES
246

TOTAL FAT
10g

SATURATED FAT
1g

CHOLESTEROL
1mg

SODIUM
387mg

CARBS
32g

DIETARY FIBER
4g

PROTEIN
9g

DIETARY EXCHANGES

2 bread/starch, 1 meat, 1 fat

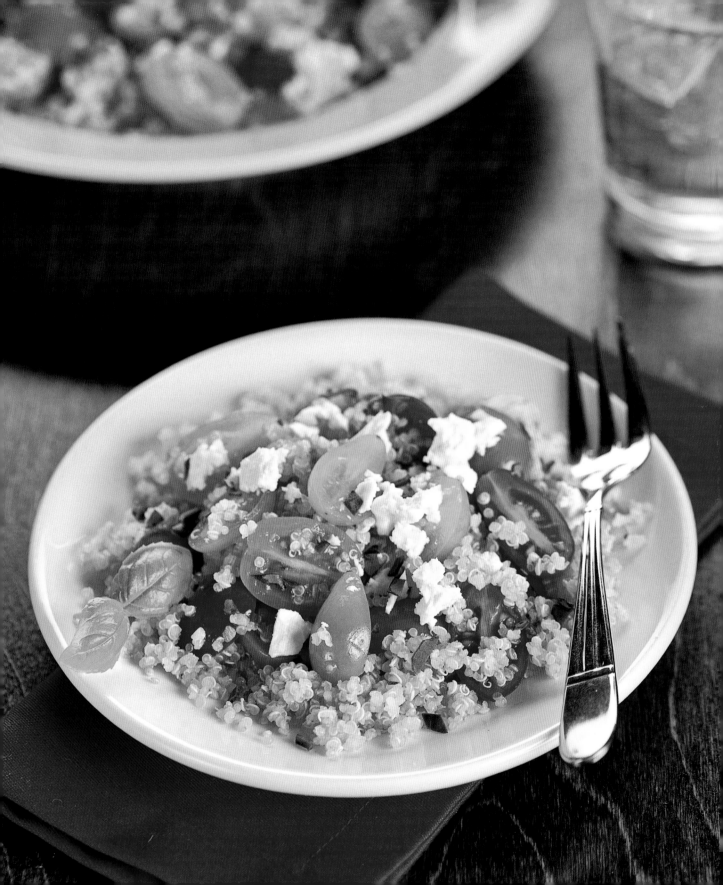

SPINACH SALAD WITH POMEGRANATE VINAIGRETTE

MAKES 4 SERVINGS

- 1 package (5 ounces) baby spinach
- ½ cup pomegranate seeds (arils)
- ¼ cup crumbled goat cheese
- 2 tablespoons chopped walnuts, toasted*
- ¼ cup pomegranate juice
- 2 tablespoons olive oil
- 1 tablespoon red wine vinegar
- 1 tablespoon honey
- ¼ teaspoon salt
- ¼ teaspoon black pepper

To toast walnuts, spread in single layer in heavy-bottomed skillet. Cook over medium heat 1 to 2 minutes, stirring frequently, until nuts are lightly browned. Remove from skillet immediately. Cool before using.

1. Combine spinach, pomegranate seeds, goat cheese and walnuts in large bowl.

2. Whisk pomegranate juice, oil, vinegar, honey, salt and pepper in small bowl until well blended. Pour over salad; gently toss to coat. Serve immediately.

Tip

For easier removal of pomegranate seeds, cut a pomegranate into pieces and immerse in a bowl of cold water. The membrane that holds the seeds in place will float to the top; discard it and collect the seeds. For convenience, you can find containers of ready-to-use pomegranate seeds in the refrigerated produce section of some supermarkets.

PER SERVING

CALORIES
161

TOTAL FAT
11g

SATURATED FAT
3g

CHOLESTEROL
4mg

SODIUM
210mg

CARBS
12g

DIETARY FIBER
1g

PROTEIN
4g

DIETARY EXCHANGES

2 vegetable, 2½ fat

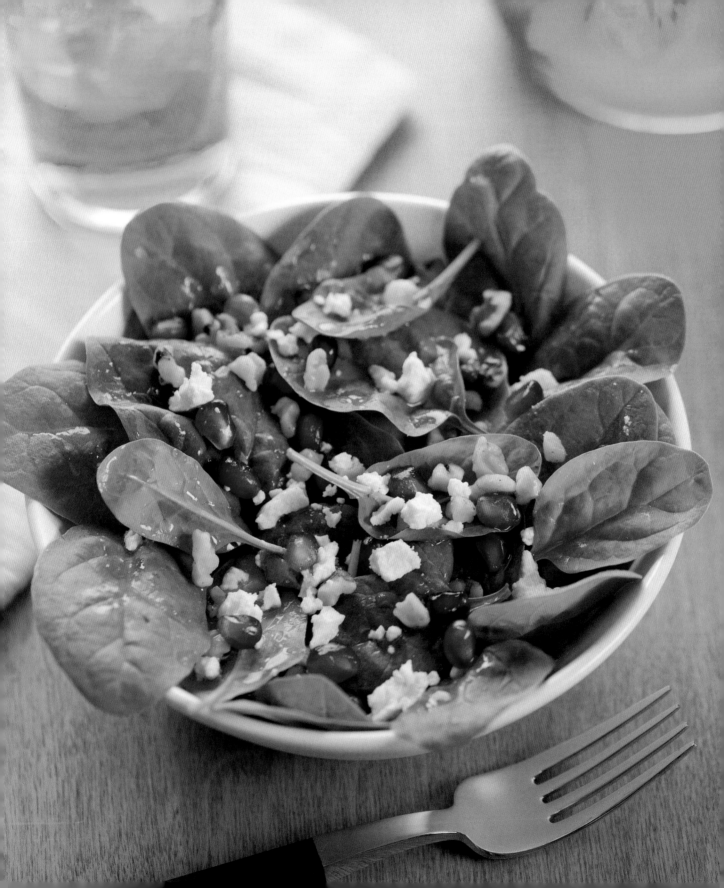

CHICKEN SATAY SALAD

MAKES 4 SERVINGS

¼ cup plus 2 tablespoons peanut sauce, divided

2 tablespoons lime juice

1 tablespoon unseasoned rice vinegar

3 teaspoons toasted sesame oil, divided

1 pound chicken tenders, cut in half lengthwise

4 cups chopped romaine lettuce

1 red bell pepper, thinly sliced

1 cup shredded carrots

1 cup sliced Persian cucumbers*

¼ cup chopped fresh cilantro

1 tablespoon peanuts, chopped

Persian cucumbers are similar to English cucumbers; they have fewer seeds and contain less water than traditional cucumbers, which gives them a sweeter flavor and crunchier texture.

1. Whisk ¼ cup peanut sauce, lime juice, vinegar and 1 teaspoon oil in large bowl until smooth and well blended. Set aside.

2. Heat remaining 2 teaspoons oil in large nonstick skillet over medium-high heat. Add chicken; cook and stir 4 minutes or until chicken is no longer pink. Remove from heat. Add remaining 2 tablespoons peanut sauce; gently toss to coat evenly.

3. Add lettuce, bell pepper, carrots and cucumbers to dressing in large bowl; toss to coat.

4. Divide salad evenly among 4 plates. Top with chicken, cilantro and peanuts.

PER SERVING

CALORIES
265

TOTAL FAT
10g

SATURATED FAT
1g

CHOLESTEROL
59mg

SODIUM
643mg

CARBS
14g

DIETARY FIBER
3g

PROTEIN
28g

DIETARY EXCHANGES

½ bread/starch, 3 meat, 1 vegetable, 1 fat

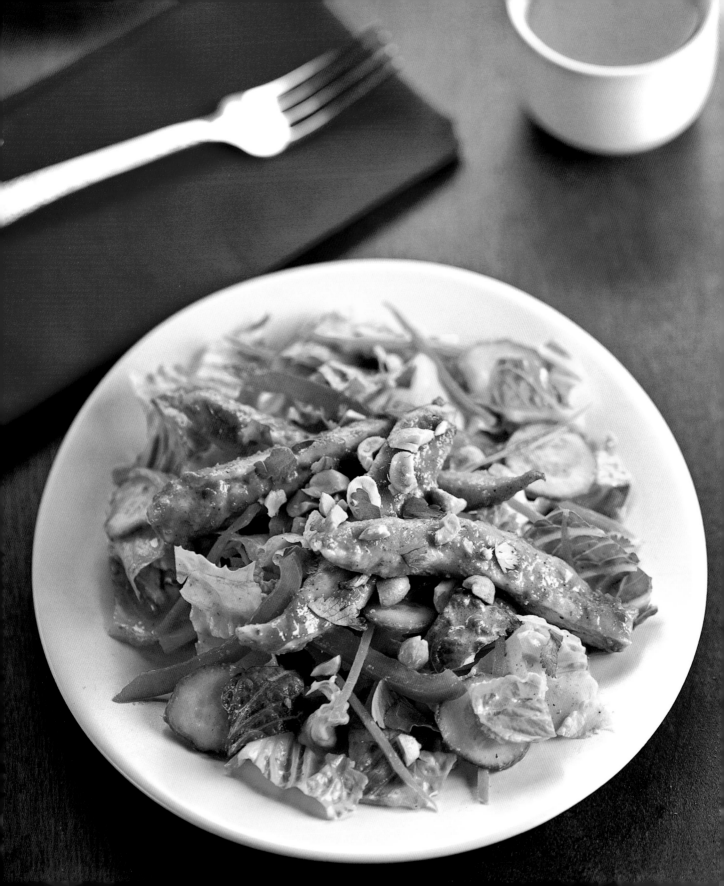

CARROT RAISIN SALAD WITH CITRUS DRESSING

MAKES 8 SERVINGS

¾ cup light sour cream

¼ cup fat-free (skim) milk

1 tablespoon honey

1 tablespoon lime juice

1 tablespoon thawed frozen orange juice concentrate

Grated peel of 1 medium orange

¼ teaspoon salt

8 medium carrots, peeled and coarsely shredded (about 2 cups)

¼ cup raisins

⅓ cup chopped cashew nuts

1. Whisk sour cream, milk, honey, lime juice, orange juice concentrate, orange peel and salt in small bowl until smooth and well blended.

2. Combine carrots and raisins in large bowl. Add dressing; toss to coat. Cover and refrigerate 30 minutes. Gently toss before serving. Top with cashews.

PER SERVING

CALORIES
127

TOTAL FAT
5g

SATURATED FAT
2g

CHOLESTEROL
8mg

SODIUM
119mg

CARBS
19g

DIETARY FIBER
3g

PROTEIN
4g

DIETARY EXCHANGES

1 vegetable, 1 fruit, 1 fat

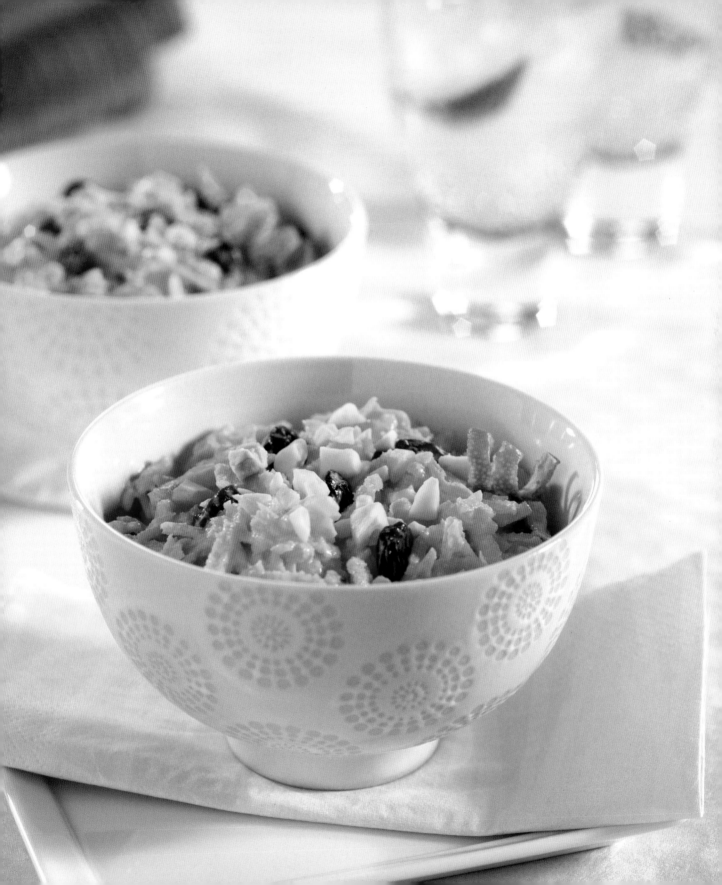

CHOPPED ROASTED CHICKEN SALAD

MAKES 4 SERVINGS

- 2 cloves garlic, minced
- 1 teaspoon dried basil
- 1 teaspoon balsamic vinegar
- ¼ teaspoon red pepper flakes
- 2 boneless skinless chicken breasts (3 ounces each)
- 6 cups chopped romaine lettuce
- 3 cups chopped baby arugula
- ½ cup chopped red cabbage
- ½ cup halved red grape tomatoes
- ½ cup chopped red bell peppers
- ½ cup sliced red onion
- ½ cup low-fat balsamic vinaigrette dressing

1. Preheat oven to 400°F. Place wire rack on rimmed baking sheet.

2. Combine garlic, basil, vinegar and red pepper flakes in small bowl. Brush mixture over each chicken breast. Place chicken on wire rack. Roast 25 to 30 minutes or until no longer pink in center. Let stand until cool enough to handle. Chop chicken.

3. Combine lettuce, arugula, red cabbage, tomatoes, bell pepper, onion and chicken in large serving bowl. Serve with dressing.

PER SERVING

CALORIES
120

TOTAL FAT
2.5g

SATURATED FAT
0g

CHOLESTEROL
30mg

SODIUM
400mg

CARBS
16g

DIETARY FIBER
3g

PROTEIN
12g

DIETARY EXCHANGES

½ bread/starch,
1½ meat,
2 vegetable

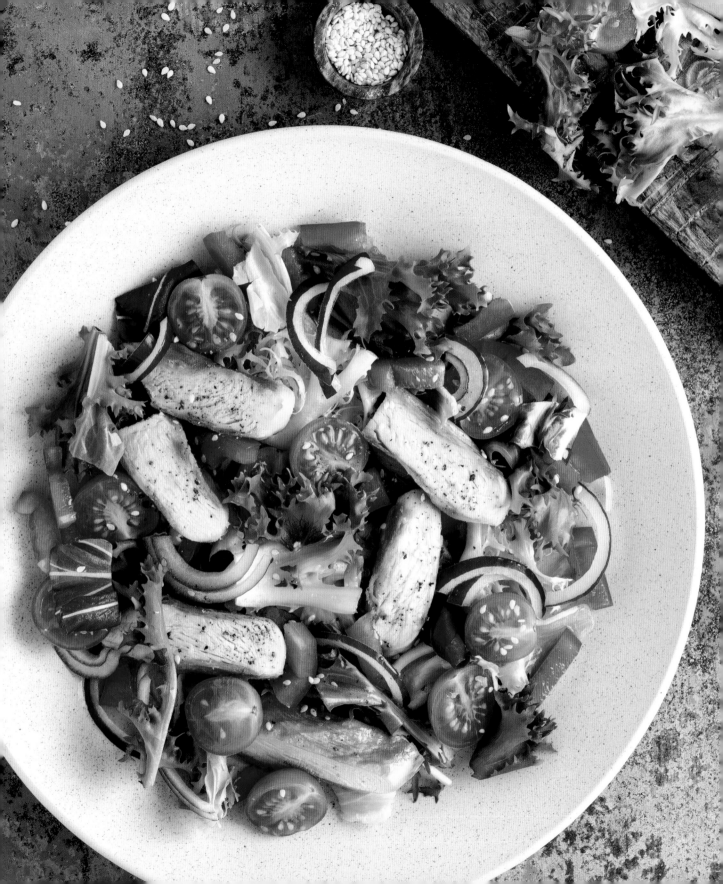

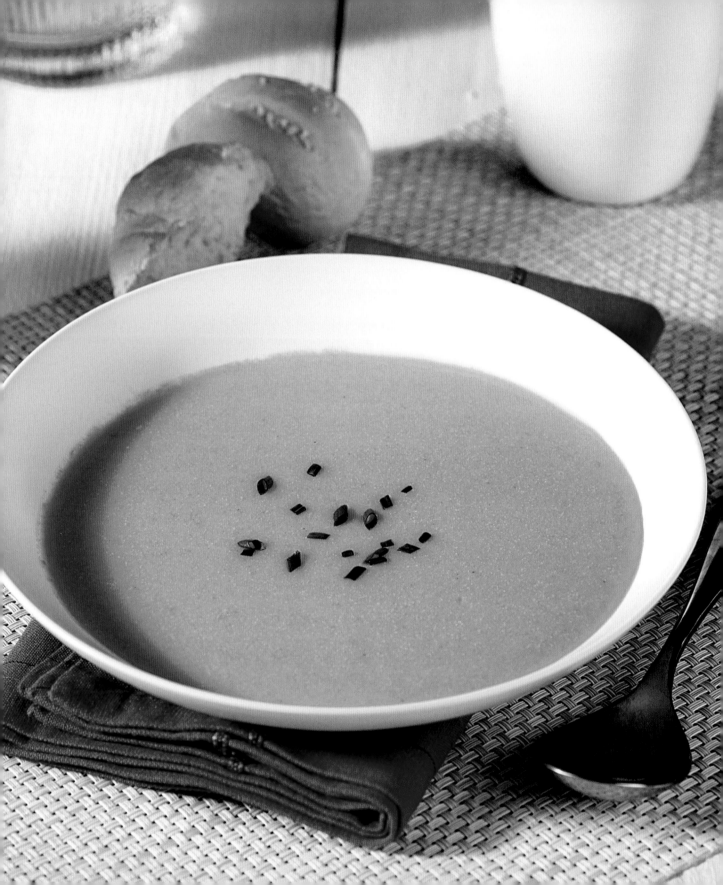

SOUPS & CHILIS

SWEET POTATO BISQUE

MAKES 4 SERVINGS

- 1 **pound sweet potatoes, peeled and cut into 2-inch chunks**
- 2 **teaspoons butter**
- ½ **cup finely chopped onion**
- 1 **teaspoon curry powder**
- ½ **teaspoon ground coriander**
- ¼ **teaspoon salt**
- ⅔ **cup unsweetened apple juice**
- 1 **cup buttermilk**
- ¼ **cup water (optional)**
  Snipped fresh chives (optional)
  Plain nonfat yogurt (optional)

1. Place sweet potatoes in large saucepan; cover with water. Bring to a boil over high heat. Cook 15 minutes or until potatoes are fork-tender. Drain; cool under cold running water.

2. Meanwhile, melt butter in small saucepan over medium heat. Add onion; cook and stir 2 minutes. Add curry powder, coriander and salt; cook and stir 1 minute or until onion is tender. Remove from heat; stir in apple juice.

3. Combine sweet potatoes, buttermilk and onion mixture in food processor or blender; process until smooth. Return to large saucepan; stir in ¼ cup water, if necessary, to thin to desired consistency. Cook and stir over medium heat until heated through. *Do not boil.* Garnish with chives or dollop of yogurt.

PER SERVING

CALORIES
160

TOTAL FAT
3g

SATURATED FAT
1g

CHOLESTEROL
2mg

SODIUM
231mg

CARBS
31g

DIETARY FIBER
4g

PROTEIN
4g

DIETARY EXCHANGES

1½ bread/starch, ½ fruit, ½ fat

EGG DROP SOUP

MAKES 2 SERVINGS

- 2 cans (about 14 ounces each) fat-free reduced-sodium chicken broth
- 1 tablespoon reduced-sodium soy sauce
- 2 teaspoons cornstarch
- ½ cup cholesterol-free egg substitute
- ¼ cup thinly sliced green onions

1. Bring broth to a boil in large saucepan over high heat. Reduce heat to medium-low.

2. Whisk soy sauce and cornstarch in small bowl until smooth and well blended; stir into broth. Cook and stir 2 minutes or until slightly thickened.

3. Stirring constantly in one direction, slowly pour egg substitute in thin stream into soup.

4. Ladle soup into bowls; sprinkle with green onions.

PER SERVING

CALORIES
45

TOTAL FAT
1g

SATURATED FAT
1g

CHOLESTEROL
0mg

SODIUM
243mg

CARBS
3g

DIETARY FIBER
1g

PROTEIN
7g

DIETARY EXCHANGES

1 meat

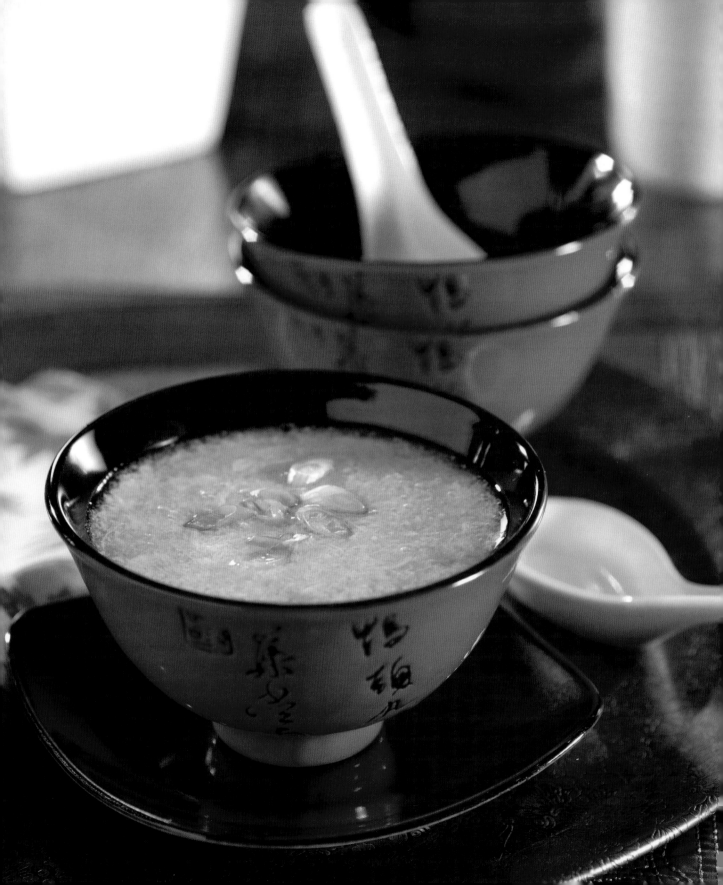

LENTIL CHILI

MAKES 5 SERVINGS

- 1 tablespoon canola oil
- 4 cloves garlic, minced
- 1 tablespoon chili powder
- 1 package (32 ounces) reduced-sodium vegetable broth
- ¾ cup dried brown or green lentils, rinsed and sorted
- 2 teaspoons smoked chipotle hot pepper sauce
- 2 cups peeled diced butternut squash
- 1 can (about 14 ounces) no-salt-added diced tomatoes
- ½ cup chopped fresh cilantro
- ¼ cup pepitas (pumpkin seeds) (optional)

1. Heat oil in large saucepan over medium heat. Add garlic; cook and stir 1 minute. Stir in chili powder; cook and stir 30 seconds.

2. Add broth, lentils and hot pepper sauce; bring to a boil over high heat. Reduce heat to low; simmer 15 minutes. Stir in squash and tomatoes; continue simmering 18 to 20 minutes or until lentils and squash are tender.

3. Ladle into bowls; top with cilantro and pepitas, if desired.

Note

Lentils are not only a good source of iron and protein, but are packed with dietary fiber. The soluble fiber in lentils helps to stabilize blood sugar levels while the insoluble fiber is known to lower high cholesterol levels and promote digestive health. Pepitas add a nice crunch to the meal for an additional 36 calories, 3 grams of fat, 2 grams of protein, and less than 1 gram of carbohydrate (for 2½ teaspoons). They're a good source of plant sterols, which have been found to promote heart health.

PER SERVING

CALORIES
184

TOTAL FAT
3g

SATURATED FAT
1g

CHOLESTEROL
0mg

SODIUM
322mg

CARBS
32g

DIETARY FIBER
12g

PROTEIN
10g

DIETARY EXCHANGES

2 bread/starch, 1 meat

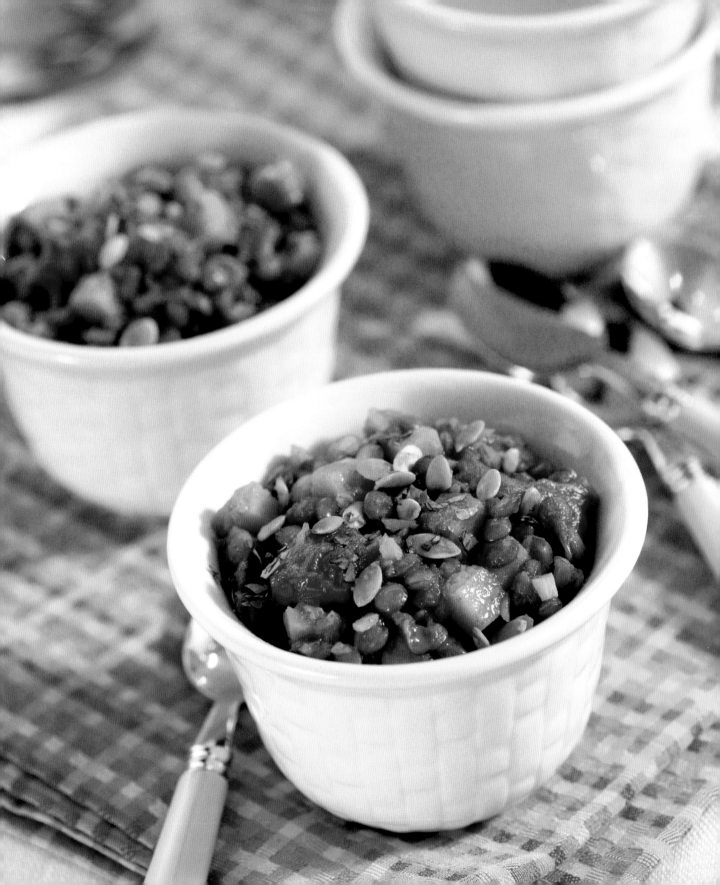

SLOW COOKER VEGGIE STEW

MAKES 4 SERVINGS

- 1 tablespoon vegetable oil
- ⅔ cup carrot slices
- ½ cup diced onion
- 2 cloves garlic, chopped
- 2 cans (about 14 ounces each) vegetable broth
- 1½ cups chopped green cabbage
- ½ cup cut green beans
- ½ cup diced zucchini
- 1 tablespoon tomato paste
- ½ teaspoon dried basil
- ½ teaspoon dried oregano
- ¼ teaspoon salt

Slow Cooker Directions

1. Heat oil in medium skillet over medium-high heat. Add carrot, onion and garlic; cook and stir until tender. Transfer to slow cooker.

2. Stir in remaining ingredients. Cover; cook on LOW 8 to 10 hours or on HIGH 4 to 5 hours.

PER SERVING

CALORIES
80

TOTAL FAT
3.5g

SATURATED FAT
0.5g

CHOLESTEROL
0mg

SODIUM
370mg

CARBS
11g

DIETARY FIBER
3g

PROTEIN
2g

DIETARY EXCHANGES

2 vegetable, 1 fat

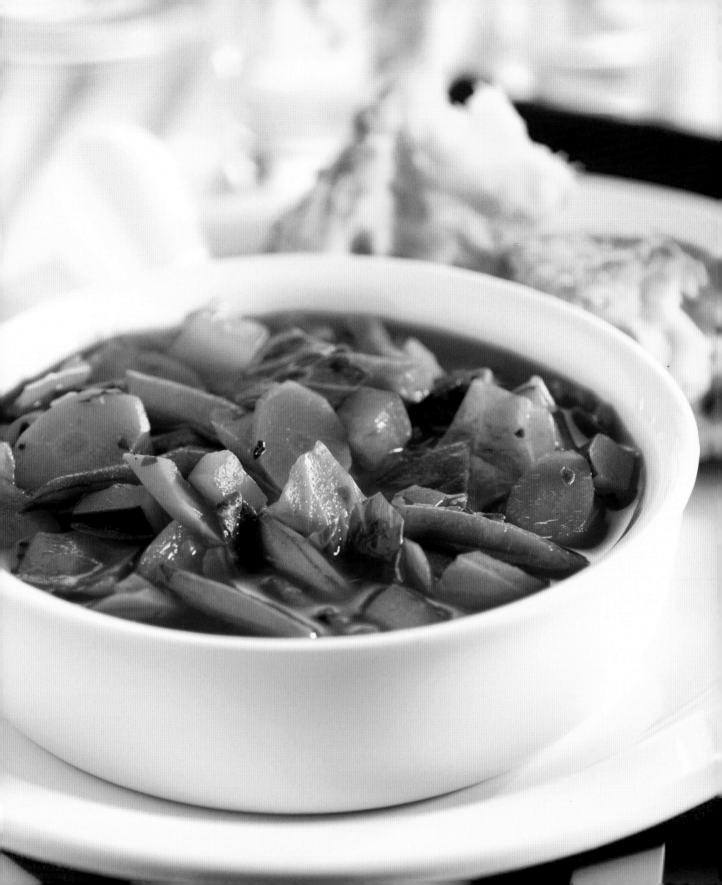

CURRIED CREAMY SWEET POTATO SOUP

MAKES 4 SERVINGS

4 cups water

1 pound sweet potatoes, peeled and cut into 1-inch cubes

1 tablespoon plus 1 teaspoon butter or margarine, divided

2 cups finely chopped yellow onions

2 cups fat-free (skim) milk, divided

¾ teaspoon curry powder

½ teaspoon salt

Dash ground red pepper (optional)

1. Bring water to a boil in large saucepan over high heat. Add potatoes; return to a boil. Reduce heat to medium-low and simmer, uncovered, 15 minutes or until potatoes are tender.

2. Meanwhile, heat medium nonstick skillet over medium-high heat until hot. Coat with nonstick cooking spray; add 1 teaspoon butter and tilt skillet to coat bottom. Add onions; cook 8 minutes or until tender and golden.

3. Drain potatoes; place in blender with onions, 1 cup milk, curry powder, salt and ground red pepper, if desired. Blend until completely smooth. Return potato mixture to saucepan and stir in remaining 1 cup milk. Cook 5 minutes over medium-high heat or until heated through. Remove from heat and stir in remaining 1 tablespoon butter.

PER SERVING

CALORIES
201

TOTAL FAT
5g

SATURATED FAT
3g

CHOLESTEROL
13mg

SODIUM
406mg

CARBS
35g

DIETARY FIBER
4g

PROTEIN
7g

DIETARY EXCHANGES

2 bread/starch, 1 vegetable, 1 fat

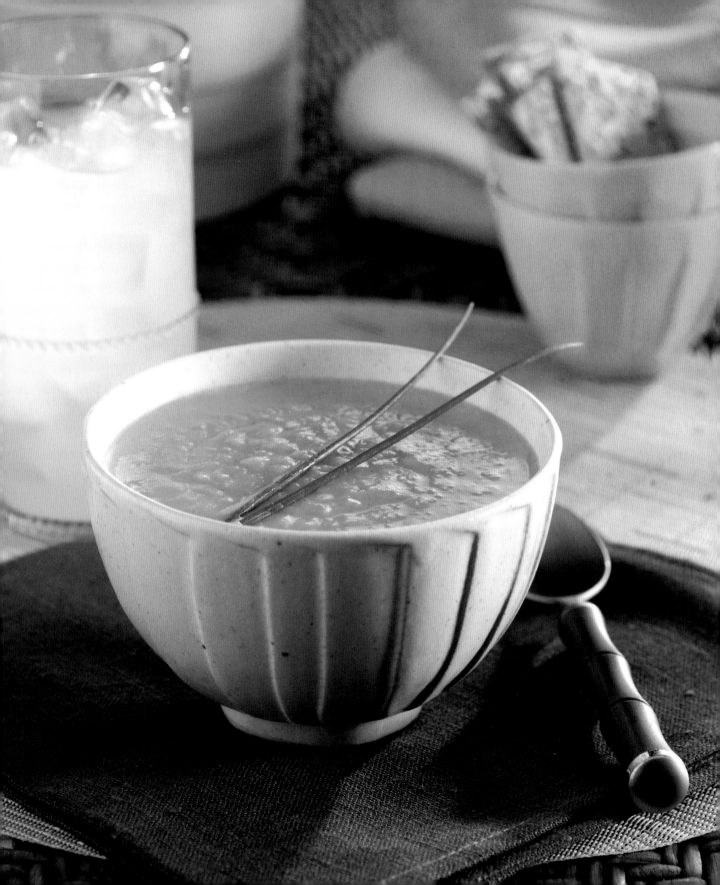

BLACK AND WHITE CHILI

MAKES 6 SERVINGS

1 pound chicken tenders, cut into ¾-inch pieces

1 cup coarsely chopped onion

1 can (about 15 ounces) Great Northern beans, drained

1 can (about 15 ounces) black beans, drained

1 can (about 14 ounces) Mexican-style stewed tomatoes, undrained

2 tablespoons Texas-style chili powder seasoning mix

Slow Cooker Directions

1. Spray large skillet with nonstick cooking spray; heat over medium heat until hot. Add chicken and onion; cook and stir 5 minutes or until chicken is browned.

2. Combine chicken mixture, beans, tomatoes with juice and chili seasoning in slow cooker. Cover; cook on LOW 4 to 4½ hours.

Serving Suggestion

For a change of pace, this delicious chili is excellent served over cooked rice or pasta.

PER SERVING

CALORIES
260

TOTAL FAT
2g

SATURATED FAT
1g

CHOLESTEROL
44mg

SODIUM
403mg

CARBS
34g

DIETARY FIBER
8g

PROTEIN
27g

DIETARY EXCHANGES

2 bread/starch, 2 meat

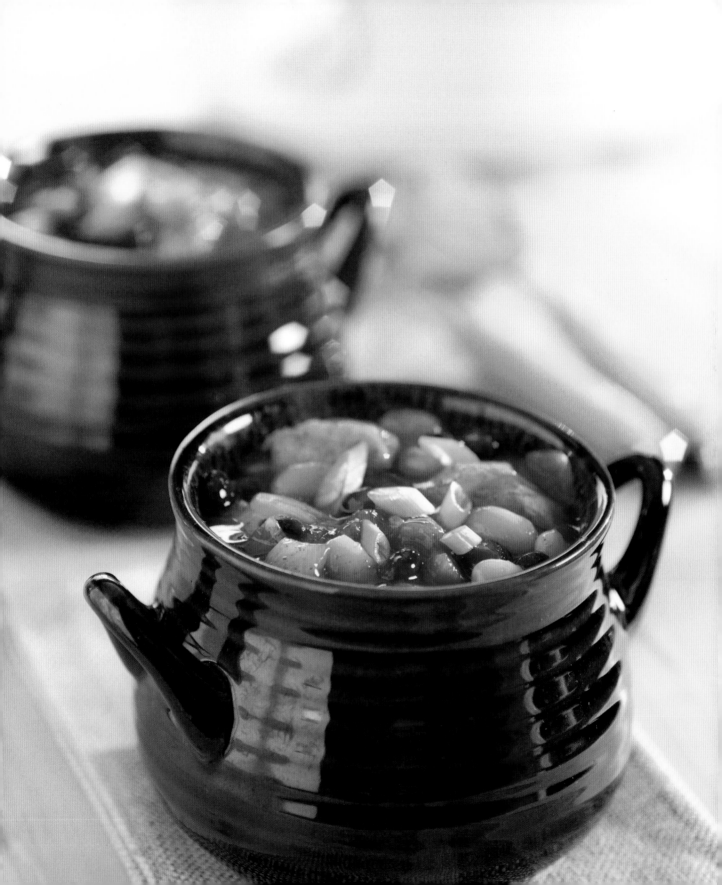

CHICKPEA-VEGETABLE SOUP

MAKES 4 SERVINGS

- 1 teaspoon olive oil
- 1 cup chopped onion
- ½ cup chopped green bell pepper
- 2 cloves garlic, minced
- 2 cans (about 14 ounces each) no-salt-added chopped tomatoes
- 3 cups water
- 2 cups broccoli florets
- 1 can (about 15 ounces) chickpeas, rinsed, drained and slightly mashed
- ½ cup (3 ounces) uncooked orzo or rosamarina pasta
- 1 bay leaf
- 1 tablespoon chopped fresh thyme *or* 1 teaspoon dried thyme
- 1 tablespoon chopped fresh rosemary *or* 1 teaspoon dried rosemary
- 1 tablespoon lime or lemon juice
- ½ teaspoon ground turmeric
- ¼ teaspoon salt
- ¼ teaspoon ground red pepper
- ¼ cup pepitas (pumpkin seeds) or sunflower kernels

1. Heat oil in large saucepan over medium heat. Add onion, bell pepper and garlic; cook and stir 5 minutes or until vegetables are tender.

2. Add tomatoes, water, broccoli, chickpeas, orzo, bay leaf, thyme, rosemary, lime juice, turmeric, salt and ground red pepper. Bring to a boil over high heat. Reduce heat to medium-low; cover and simmer 10 to 12 minutes or until orzo is tender.

3. Remove and discard bay leaf. Ladle soup into 4 serving bowls; sprinkle with pepitas.

PER SERVING

CALORIES
300

TOTAL FAT
6g

SATURATED FAT
1g

CHOLESTEROL
0mg

SODIUM
280mg

CARBS
48g

DIETARY FIBER
9g

PROTEIN
13g

DIETARY EXCHANGES

2 bread/starch, 3 vegetable, 1 fat

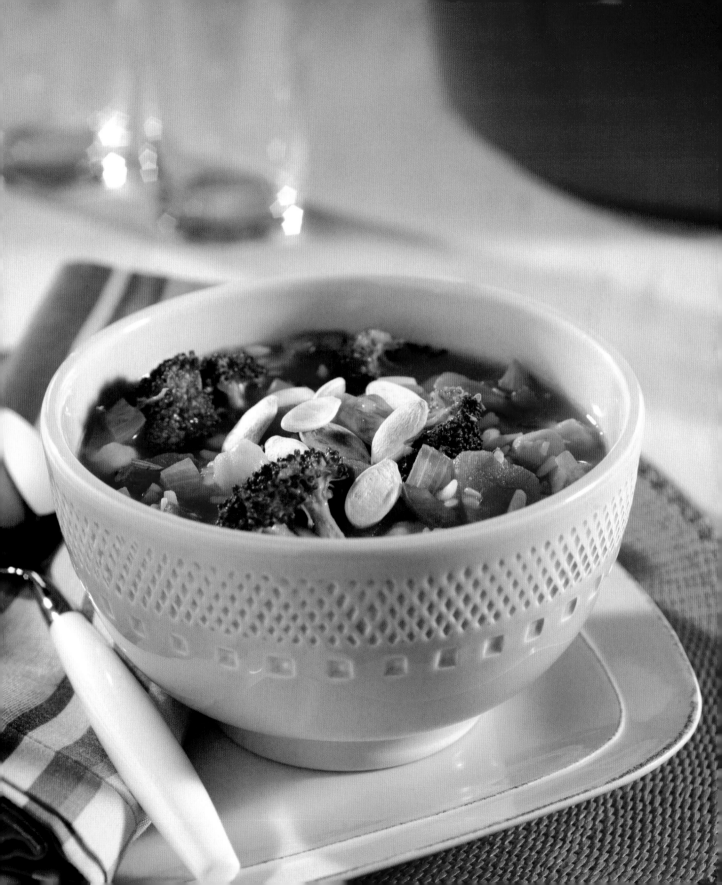

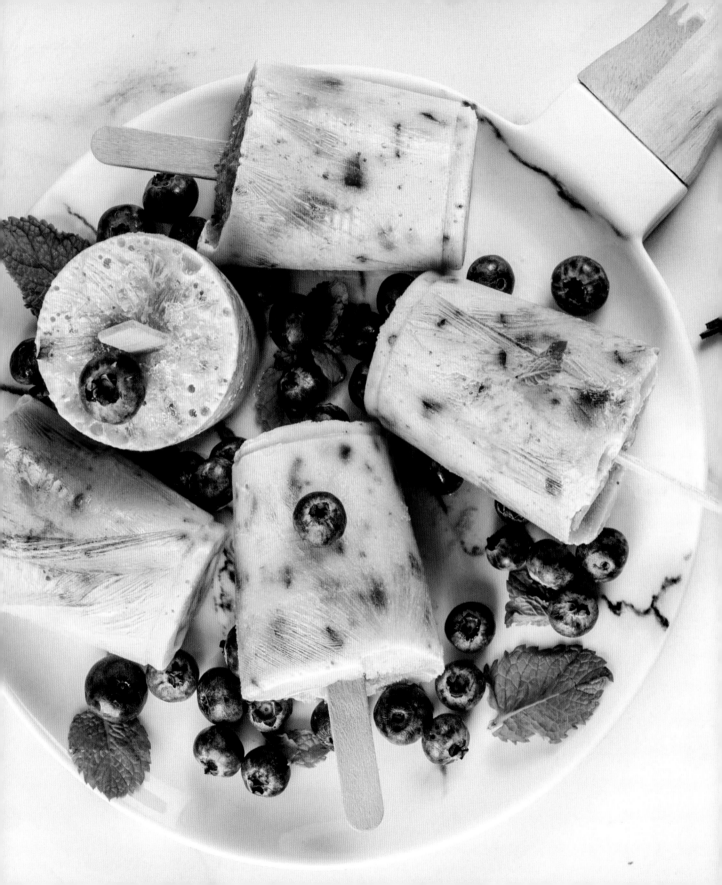

SWEET ENDINGS

FROZEN BERRY POPS

MAKES 4 POPS

1¼ cups plain nonfat Greek yogurt

¼ cup fat-free (skim) milk

2 tablespoons sugar

6 teaspoons lemon juice

1 cup chopped blueberries or raspberries

4 (5-ounce) paper or plastic cups or pop molds

4 pop sticks

1. Combine yogurt, milk, sugar and lemon juice in blender or food processor; blend until smooth. Gently stir in blueberries.

2. Pour mixture into cups. Cover top of each cup with small piece of foil. Insert sticks through center of foil. Freeze 4 hours or until firm.

3. To serve, remove foil and peel away paper cups or gently twist frozen pops out of plastic cups.

PER SERVING

CALORIES
120

TOTAL FAT
3.5g

SATURATED FAT
2.5g

CHOLESTEROL
10mg

SODIUM
30mg

CARBS
16g

DIETARY FIBER
1g

PROTEIN
7g

DIETARY EXCHANGES

½ fruit, ½ milk, ½ fat

ROCKY ROAD PUDDING

MAKES 6 SERVINGS

5 tablespoons unsweetened cocoa powder

¼ cup granulated sugar

3 tablespoons cornstarch

⅛ teaspoon salt

2½ cups low-fat (1%) milk

2 egg yolks, beaten

2 teaspoons vanilla

6 packets sugar substitute *or* equivalent of ¼ cup sugar

1 cup mini marshmallows

¼ cup chopped walnuts, toasted*

*To toast walnuts, spread in single layer in heavy skillet. Cook over medium heat 3 minutes or until nuts are fragrant, stirring frequently.

1. Combine cocoa, granulated sugar, cornstarch and salt in small saucepan; stir until well blended. Stir in milk until smooth. Cook over medium-high heat about 10 minutes or until mixture thickens and begins to boil, stirring constantly.

2. Whisk ½ cup hot milk mixture into beaten egg yolks in small bowl. Pour mixture back into saucepan; cook over medium heat 10 minutes or until mixture reaches 160°F, whisking constantly. Remove from heat; stir in vanilla.

3. Place plastic wrap on surface of pudding. Refrigerate about 20 minutes or until slightly cooled. Stir in sugar substitute. Spoon pudding into 6 dessert dishes; top with marshmallows and walnuts.

PER SERVING

CALORIES
190

TOTAL FAT
6g

SATURATED FAT
1g

CHOLESTEROL
75mg

SODIUM
121mg

CARBS
28g

DIETARY FIBER
1g

PROTEIN
7g

DIETARY EXCHANGES

1 bread/starch, ½ milk, 1 fat

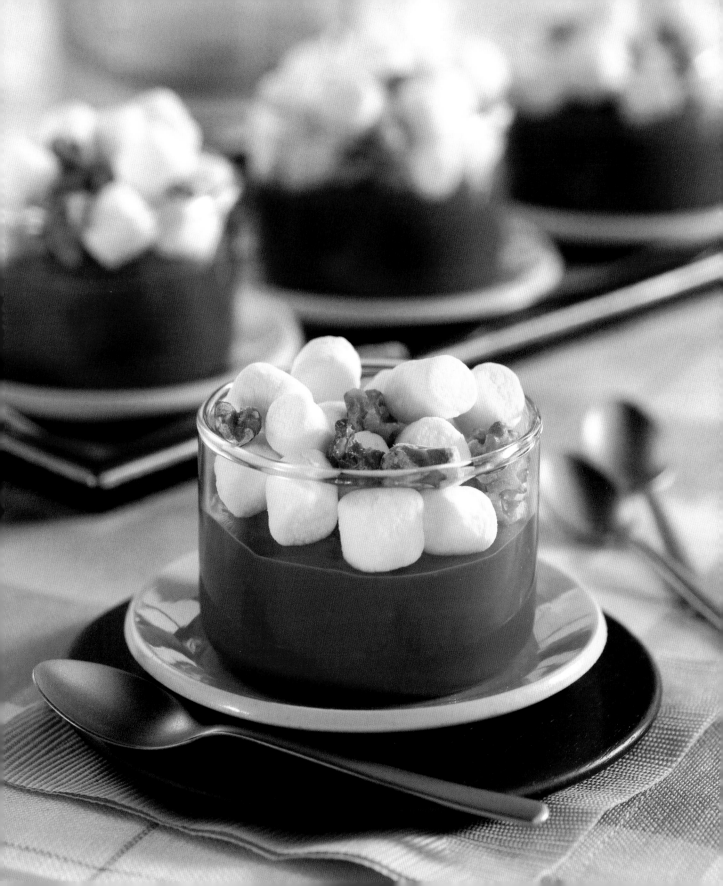

PEACH-MELBA SHORTCAKES

MAKES 4 SERVINGS

1 cup reduced-fat biscuit baking mix

¼ cup fat-free (skim) milk

2 tablespoons sugar

1¼ cups fresh raspberries

1 cup diced peeled peaches

2 tablespoons raspberry fruit spread

4 tablespoons thawed frozen whipped topping

1. Preheat oven to 425°F. Stir baking mix, milk and sugar in small bowl until smooth and well blended. Drop about 3 tablespoons per biscuit onto ungreased baking sheet. Bake 10 to 12 minutes or until tops are slightly browned. Cool on baking sheet 5 minutes.

2. Meanwhile, combine raspberries and peaches in medium bowl; set aside.

3. Microwave fruit spread in small microwavable bowl on HIGH 15 seconds or until softened.

4. Slice warm biscuits in half. Arrange biscuit bottoms on 4 serving plates. Drizzle ½ teaspoon fruit spread over each biscuit bottom. Top evenly with raspberries and peaches. Replace biscuit tops. Drizzle each shortcake with 1 teaspoon fruit spread; top with 1 tablespoon whipped topping.

PER SERVING

CALORIES
205

TOTAL FAT
3g

SATURATED FAT
1g

CHOLESTEROL
0mg

SODIUM
335mg

CARBS
42g

DIETARY FIBER
4g

PROTEIN
4g

DIETARY EXCHANGES

2 bread/starch, 1 fruit

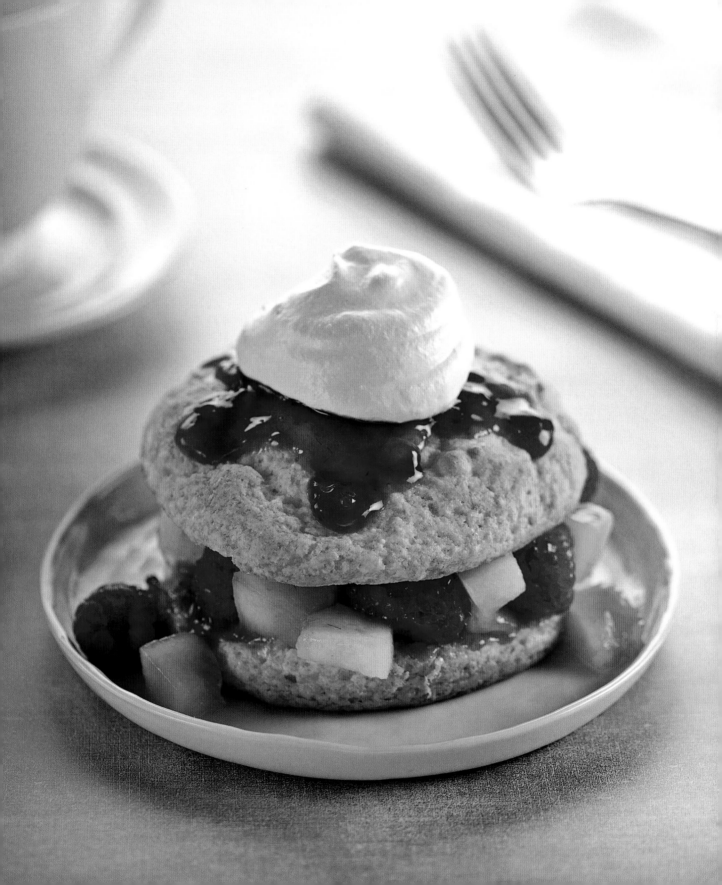

CHOCOLATE COOKIE PARFAITS

MAKES 4 SERVINGS

- 1 package (4-serving size) chocolate fat-free sugar-free instant pudding and pie filling mix
- 2 cups fat-free (skim) milk
- 8 tablespoons thawed reduced-fat whipped topping
- 4 sugar-free chocolate sandwich cookies, finely crushed
- 4 teaspoons multi-colored sprinkles

1. Prepare pudding according to package directions using 2 cups milk.

2. Spoon half of pudding into 4 parfait glasses. Spread 1 tablespoon whipped topping over pudding in each glass. Sprinkle with half of crushed cookies. Layer remaining pudding over top of cookies. Top with remaining whipped topping, cookies and sprinkles.

PER SERVING

CALORIES
158

TOTAL FAT
6g

SATURATED FAT
2g

CHOLESTEROL
2mg

SODIUM
387mg

CARBS
24g

DIETARY FIBER
0g

PROTEIN
6g

DIETARY EXCHANGES

1 bread/starch, ½ milk, 1 fat

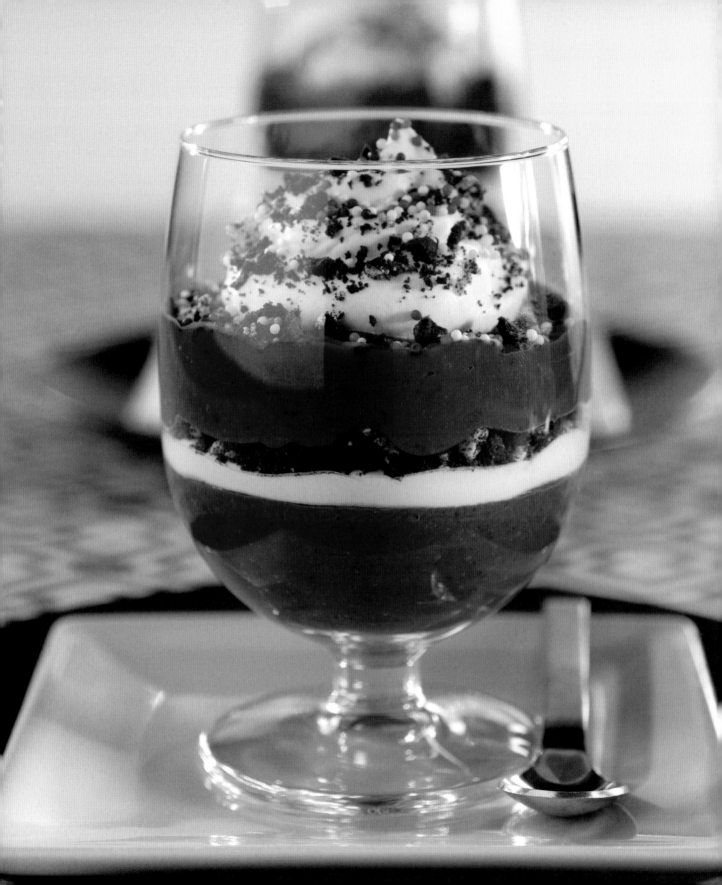

STRAWBERRY CHEESECAKE PARFAITS

MAKES 4 SERVINGS

1½ cups vanilla nonfat Greek yogurt

½ cup whipped cream cheese, at room temperature

2 tablespoons powdered sugar

1 teaspoon vanilla

2 cups sliced fresh strawberries

2 teaspoons granulated sugar

8 honey graham cracker squares, coarsely crumbled (about 2 cups)

Fresh mint leaves (optional)

1. Whisk yogurt, cream cheese, powdered sugar and vanilla in small bowl until smooth and well blended.

2. Combine strawberries and granulated sugar in small bowl; gently toss.

3. Layer ¼ cup yogurt mixture, ¼ cup strawberries and ¼ cup graham cracker crumbs in each of 4 dessert dishes. Repeat layers. Garnish with mint. Serve immediately.

PER SERVING

CALORIES
220

TOTAL FAT
7g

SATURATED FAT
3g

CHOLESTEROL
15mg

SODIUM
200mg

CARBS
29g

DIETARY FIBER
2g

PROTEIN
11g

DIETARY EXCHANGES

1 bread/starch, 1 fruit, 1 fat

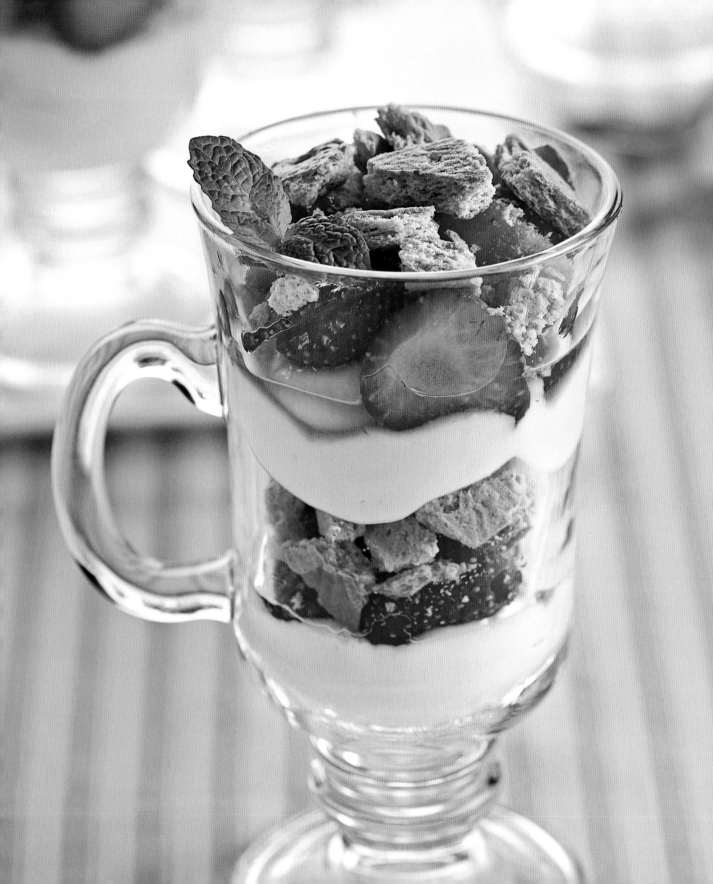

RUSTIC APPLE TART

MAKES 8 SERVINGS

1 refrigerated pie crust (half of 14-ounce package)

4 medium Granny Smith apples, peeled, cored and thinly sliced (about 4 cups)

2 tablespoons packed brown sugar

¼ teaspoon ground cinnamon

1 egg white

3 tablespoons apricot fruit spread

1. Preheat oven to 375°F. Line baking sheet with parchment paper; spray with nonstick cooking spray.

2. Roll out pie crust on lightly floured surface to 12-inch circle. Place on prepared baking sheet.

3. Combine apples, brown sugar and cinnamon in large bowl; toss to coat evenly. Arrange apples in center of pie crust to within 1 inch of edge. Fold crust over apples. Brush with egg white.

4. Bake 25 minutes. Dot with fruit spread. Bake 5 to 10 minutes or until apples are crisp-tender and crust is golden brown. Let stand 5 minutes before cutting. Serve warm.

PER SERVING

CALORIES
160

TOTAL FAT
6g

SATURATED FAT
2g

CHOLESTEROL
3mg

SODIUM
137mg

CARBS
26g

DIETARY FIBER
1g

PROTEIN
1g

DIETARY EXCHANGES

1 bread/starch, ½ fruit, 1 fat

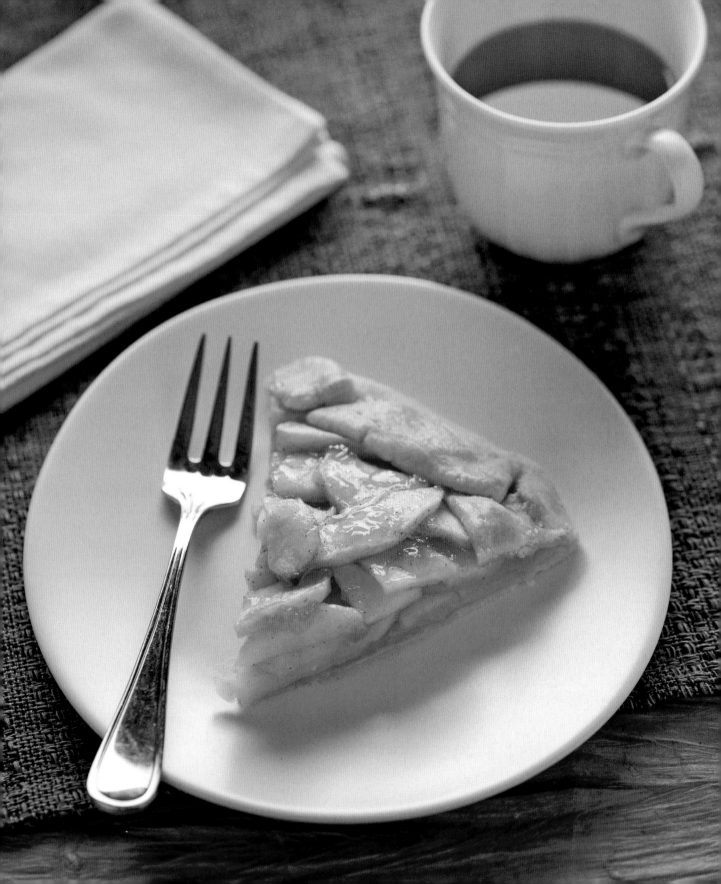

WARM OATMEAL APRICOT GINGER COOKIES

MAKES 2 DOZEN COOKIES (2 COOKIES PER SERVING)

- **3 tablespoons canola oil**
- **¼ cup cholesterol-free egg substitute**
- **1¼ cups old-fashioned rolled oats**
- **⅓ cup all-purpose flour**
- **⅓ cup granulated sugar**
- **¼ cup packed sucralose-brown sugar blend**
- **1½ teaspoons ground ginger**
- **¾ teaspoon baking soda**
- **¼ teaspoon salt**
- **6 ounces whole dried apricots, chopped**

1. Preheat oven to 375°F. Combine oil and egg substitute in medium bowl. Using an electric mixer on high speed, beat until well blended. Add remaining ingredients except apricots; reduce to medium speed, and beat until well blended. Stir in apricots.

2. Line 2 cookie sheets with parchment paper. Using a tablespoon, spoon 6 cookies on each cookie sheet. (Do not spoon more than 6 to a sheet, they will spread while baking.) Bake 6 minutes or until slightly golden on edges and light in the middle. (They will not look done at this point, but will continue to cook while cooling.) Remove from oven, let stand on cookie sheet 3 minutes before removing. Continue with remaining batter.

PER SERVING

CALORIES
160

TOTAL FAT
4g

SATURATED FAT
0g

CHOLESTEROL
0mg

SODIUM
140mg

CARBS
28g

DIETARY FIBER
2g

PROTEIN
2g

DIETARY EXCHANGES

½ bread/starch, ½ other carb, ½ fruit, 1 fat

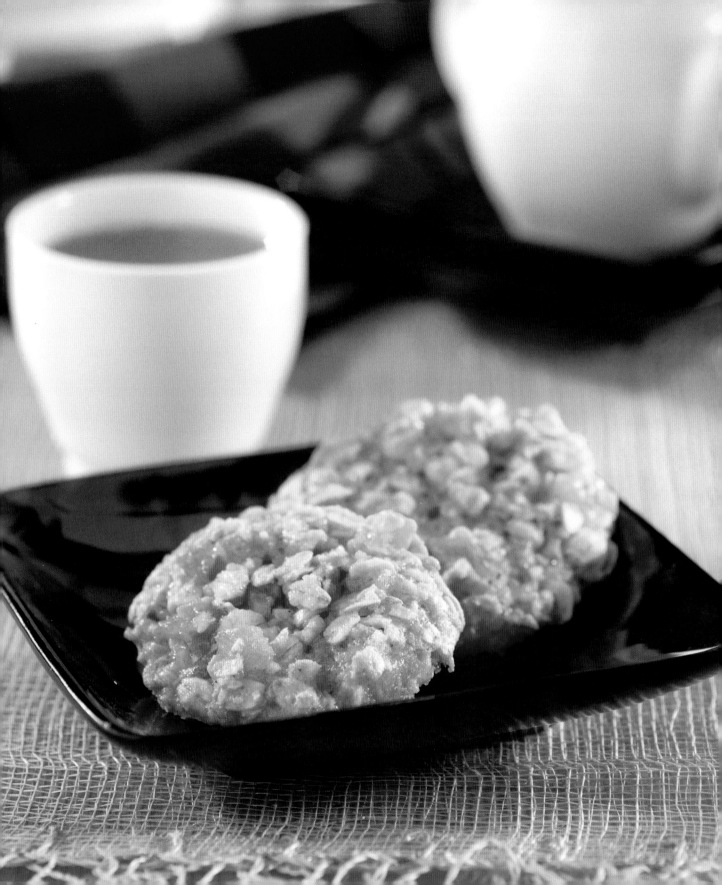

CREAMY BANANA PARFAIT WITH NUTMEG

MAKES 4 SERVINGS

1 container (6 ounces) vanilla nonfat yogurt

2 ounces reduced-fat cream cheese, softened

1¼ cups fat-free (skim) milk

¼ teaspoon vanilla

1 package (4-serving size) sugar-free instant vanilla pudding and pie filling mix

⅛ teaspoon ground nutmeg

1 ripe medium banana, very thinly sliced

½ cup (about 12) low-fat vanilla wafers, crushed

¼ cup thawed frozen fat-free whipped topping

1. Combine yogurt and cream cheese in medium bowl; beat with electric mixer at medium speed until smooth. Gradually add milk and vanilla; beat until smooth. Add pudding mix and nutmeg; beat until well blended.

2. Spoon pudding mixture into each of 4 wine goblets or parfait glasses. Top with banana slices; sprinkle with cookie crumbs. (Cover bananas evenly with cookie crumbs to prevent discoloration.)

3. Cover parfaits with plastic wrap. Refrigerate at least 1 hour or up to 4 hours before serving.

4. Top each parfait with 2 tablespoons whipped topping.

PER SERVING

CALORIES
235

TOTAL FAT
7g

SATURATED FAT
3g

CHOLESTEROL
12mg

SODIUM
658mg

CARBS
37g

DIETARY FIBER
1g

PROTEIN
7g

DIETARY EXCHANGES

2½ bread/starch, ½ fruit, ½ milk, 1 fat

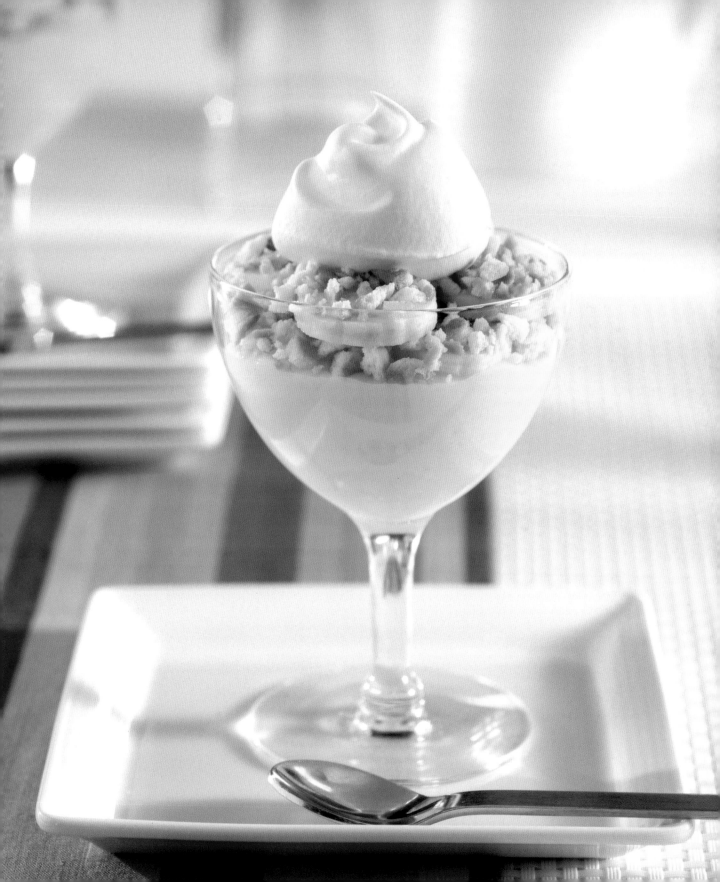

TANGY LEMON-CRANBERRY MINI CAKES

MAKES 6 CAKES (ABOUT 12 SERVINGS)

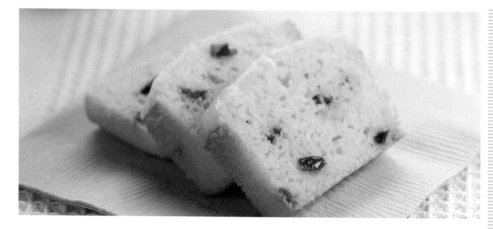

1½ **cups all-purpose flour**

¾ **teaspoon baking soda**

¾ **teaspoon baking powder**

¼ **teaspoon salt**

¾ **cup sugar**

⅔ **cup plain nonfat Greek yogurt**

½ **cup vegetable oil**

2 **eggs**

2 **egg whites**

½ **cup fresh lemon juice**

Grated peel of 2 lemons

1 **teaspoon vanilla**

½ **cup dried cranberries**

1. Preheat oven to 350°F. Spray 6 mini (4¼×2½-inch) loaf pans with nonstick cooking spray.

2. Combine flour, baking soda, baking powder and salt in medium bowl; mix well. Whisk sugar, yogurt, oil, eggs, egg whites, lemon juice, lemon peel and vanilla in large bowl until well blended. Gradually stir in flour mixture until combined. Fold in cranberries. Pour evenly into prepared pans.

3. Bake 30 minutes or until toothpick inserted into centers comes out clean. Cool 5 minutes in pans. Remove to wire racks; cool completely.

Tip

Each mini loaf pan used in this recipe holds 1 cup batter. The size of the pans may be found labeled by volume or dimension.

PER SERVING

CALORIES
230

TOTAL FAT
10g

SATURATED FAT
1g

CHOLESTEROL
0mg

SODIUM
184mg

CARBS
30g

DIETARY FIBER
1g

PROTEIN
5g

DIETARY EXCHANGES

2 bread/starch, 2 fat

METRIC CONVERSION CHART

VOLUME MEASUREMENTS (dry)

1/8 teaspoon = 0.5 mL
1/4 teaspoon = 1 mL
1/2 teaspoon = 2 mL
3/4 teaspoon = 4 mL
1 teaspoon = 5 mL
1 tablespoon = 15 mL
2 tablespoons = 30 mL
1/4 cup = 60 mL
1/3 cup = 75 mL
1/2 cup = 125 mL
2/3 cup = 150 mL
3/4 cup = 175 mL
1 cup = 250 mL
2 cups = 1 pint = 500 mL
3 cups = 750 mL
4 cups = 1 quart = 1 L

VOLUME MEASUREMENTS (fluid)

1 fluid ounce (2 tablespoons) = 30 mL
4 fluid ounces (1/2 cup) = 125 mL
8 fluid ounces (1 cup) = 250 mL
12 fluid ounces (1 1/2 cups) = 375 mL
16 fluid ounces (2 cups) = 500 mL

WEIGHTS (mass)

1/2 ounce = 15 g
1 ounce = 30 g
3 ounces = 90 g
4 ounces = 120 g
8 ounces = 225 g
10 ounces = 285 g
12 ounces = 360 g
16 ounces = 1 pound = 450 g

DIMENSIONS

1/16 inch = 2 mm
1/8 inch = 3 mm
1/4 inch = 6 mm
1/2 inch = 1.5 cm
3/4 inch = 2 cm
1 inch = 2.5 cm

OVEN TEMPERATURES

250°F = 120°C
275°F = 140°C
300°F = 150°C
325°F = 160°C
350°F = 180°C
375°F = 190°C
400°F = 200°C
425°F = 220°C
450°F = 230°C

BAKING PAN SIZES

Utensil	Size in Inches/Quarts	Metric Volume	Size in Centimeters
Baking or Cake Pan (square or rectangular)	8×8×2	2 L	20×20×5
	9×9×2	2.5 L	23×23×5
	12×8×2	3 L	30×20×5
	13×9×2	3.5 L	33×23×5
Loaf Pan	8×4×3	1.5 L	20×10×7
	9×5×3	2 L	23×13×7
Round Layer Cake Pan	8×1½	1.2 L	20×4
	9×1½	1.5 L	23×4
Pie Plate	8×1¼	750 mL	20×3
	9×1¼	1 L	23×3
Baking Dish or Casserole	1 quart	1 L	—
	1½ quart	1.5 L	—
	2 quart	2 L	—